Contents

About the author ....

Introduction 5

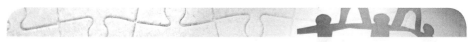

Section 1: Legislation, policies and working with offenders 7

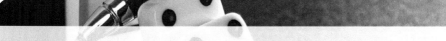

**Section 2: Active support and common mental
health problems** **32**

Section 3: Assessing risk and recording information **62**

References 79

Further reading 79

Useful contacts 81

About the author

Martin Spooner is presently working as a learning and development manager for a private company that specialises in mental health care. He is an experienced clinician and communicator, and has built his skills over his many years in practice. As well as being a registered nurse, Martin is a qualified counsellor, teacher and facilitator, and he uses these skills to empower, enable and educate, whether that is in practice or in the classroom.

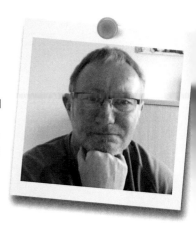

Working in Secure Forensic Mental Health Settings

A Care Quality Guide for support workers and staff

© Martin Spooner

The author has asserted his rights in accordance with the Copyright, Designs and Patents Act (1988) to be identified as the author of this work.

Published by:
Pavilion Publishing and Media Ltd
Rayford House, School Road, Hove, BN3 5HX
Tel: 01273 434 943
Fax: 01273 227 308
Email: info@pavpub.com

Published 2015.

All rights reserved. No part of this publication may be reproduced, stored in a retrieval system, or transmitted in any form or by any means, electronic, mechanical, photocopying, recording or otherwise, without prior permission in writing of the publisher and the copyright owners.

A catalogue record for this book is available from the British Library.

Print ISBN: 978-1-910366-46-2

EPUB ISBN: 978-1-910366-47-9

EPDF ISBN: 978-1-910366-48-6

MOBI ISBN: 978-1-910366-49-3

Pavilion is the leading publisher and provider of professional development products and services for workers in the health, social care, education and community safety sectors. We believe that everyone has the right to fulfil their potential and we strive to supply products and services that help raise standards, promote best practices and support continuing professional development.

Author: Martin Spooner

Editor: Catherine Ansell-Jones, Pavilion Publishing and Media Ltd

Cover design: Emma Dawe, Pavilion Publishing and Media Ltd

Layout design: Emma Dawe, Pavilion Publishing and Media Ltd

Printing: CMP Digital Print Solutions

Introduction

Working within secure forensic mental health settings can be highly demanding, and individuals starting work in this complex sector are faced with a number of challenges. This guide has been written both to support new staff members to develop their understanding of working with offenders with mental disorders, and to provide those who are already working in secure forensic settings with the opportunity to reflect on their practice.

Health and social care support workers play an essential role in providing effective, therapeutic and high quality care for those detained in secure forensic facilities. Whether they work in locked rehabilitation units, community forensic services or in low, medium or high secure facilities, they all need to gain the basic skills required to provide active support for the individuals detained in secure forensic settings.

Care Quality Guides

Pavilion's Care Quality Guides aim to help you refresh, develop or extend your learning in key areas of practice.

- If you are new to working with a particular client group or in a new role, you can use the material to quickly develop knowledge you will need, and where appropriate, work towards a relevant qualification.

- If you are a more experienced worker, you can use the guides

to refresh your learning, and to contribute towards your continuing professional development.

- If you are a manager, you can use these guides with staff to meet your responsibilities for providing induction and staff supervision, and opportunities for training and development and continuing professional development. This will contribute towards meeting Care Quality Commission (CQC) Standards.

Maintaining and improving your knowledge and skills

This guide can help towards maintaining and improving your knowledge and skills.

You can work through the guide, section by section, completing the **thinking and practice activities** as you go.

Supervision and continuing professional development (CPD)

This guide can be used for continuing professional development. If you are a manager, you might like to ask your staff members to work through it section by section, completing the **thinking and practice activities** each contains. Their responses can be discussed as part of on-going supervision, and on completion of the guide, you can both fill in the CPD certificate at the end.

Meeting the Care Quality Commission (CQC) Standards

If you are a manager or provider of a health and social care service, you can use this guide for staff development in order to contribute towards meeting current training standards and to prepare for quality checks and inspections. In particular, using this guide with your staff will contribute towards ensuring that they have training and CPD opportunities to strengthen and develop their skills and knowledge.

The National Occupational Standards

The guide will also help you to evidence aspects of the following Forensic Mental Health National Occupational Standards: Care Certificate and Diploma in Health and Social Care levels 2 and 3.

Forensic Mental Health Occupational Standards	
SFHFMH1	Assess, diagnose and formulate an individual's mental health disorder
SFHFMH3	Observe an individual who presents a significant imminent risk to themselves or others
SFHFMH8	Assess and formulate an individual's needs for forensic mental health treatment and care
SFHFMH9	Develop and review an integrated care programme for an individual in forensic mental health care
SFHFMH11	Support an individual in forensic mental health care to participate in treatment
SFHFMH12	Manage hostility and risk with non-co-operative individuals, families and carers
SFHFMH13	Help an individual to feel more psychologically secure
SFHFMH15	Increase the individual's capacity to manage negative or distressing thoughts and emotional states

Legislation, policies and working with offenders

Introduction

This section covers the Mental Health Act (2007) and how it works with the five guiding principles of the Mental Capacity Act (2005). It examines the nature and characteristics of issues faced by offenders with mental disorders and the challenges individuals can present. It explores the history of secure forensic mental health facilities and their role in keeping people safe. It also covers some important issues to consider when working with individuals.

Anyone working within a secure forensic mental health setting needs to understand the context in which care and treatment are provided. The context is complex and can include the impact on the individual being cared for and treated; the impact on the people who work within the setting; the way that visitors interact with the service and how they view the care and treatment being provided; the way that professionals work with people on a day-to-day basis; how professionals can affect the present and the future of those in their care.

Legislation and policies that support the human rights of those detained in secure forensic mental health settings

The Mental Health Act (2007) and the Mental Capacity Act (2005)

In working with people detained in secure mental health settings, it is important to understand the guiding principles of the Mental Health Act (2007) (MHA) and how they work with the five guiding principles of the Mental Capacity Act (2005) (MCA).

The Mental Health Act (2007) provides legislation for registered medical practitioners, approved clinicians, managers and approved mental health professionals. It also legislates on how doctors and other professionals provide medical treatment for mental disorders.

The Mental Capacity Act (2005) provides a statutory framework for people who lack capacity to make decisions for themselves. It sets out who can make decisions on behalf of a person who lacks capacity, in which situations and how they should go about this.

The five principles of the Mental Health Act (2007)

1. **The purpose principle:** Decisions under the act must be taken with a view to minimising the undesirable effects of mental disorder, by maximising the safety and well-being (mental and physical) of individuals, promoting their recovery and protecting other people from harm.

2. **The least restriction principle:** People taking action without an individual's consent must attempt to keep to a minimum the restrictions they impose on the person's liberty, having regard to the purpose for which the restrictions are imposed.

3. **The respect principle:** People taking decisions under the act must

recognise the diverse needs, values and circumstances of each individual, including their race, religion, culture, gender, age, sexual orientation and any disability. They must consider the person's views, wishes and feelings (whether expressed at the time or in advance), so far as they are reasonably ascertainable, and follow those wishes wherever practicable and consistent with the purpose of the decision. There must be no unlawful discrimination.

Thinking activity

How does your own practice fit in with the principles of the acts?

4. **The participation principle:** Individuals must be given the opportunity to be involved as far as is practicable in the circumstances, in planning, developing and reviewing their own treatment and care to help ensure that it is delivered in a way that is as appropriate and effective as possible. The involvement of carers, family members and other people who have an interest in the person's welfare should be encouraged (unless there are particular reasons to the contrary) and their views must be taken seriously.

5. **The effectiveness, efficiency and equity principle:** People taking decisions under the act must seek to use the resources available to them and to individuals in the most effective, efficient and equitable way, to meet people's needs and achieve the purpose for which the decision was taken. NB: Note the language of the act and how it closely mirrors other legislation, including the Equalities Act (2010) and the Mental Capacity Act (2005). If you breach one, there is a good chance that you breach them all. In the UK we also have a common law duty to protect the rights of others.

The five principles of the Mental Capacity Act (2005)

1. It must be assumed that a person has capacity unless it is established that they lack capacity.

2. A person must not be treated as unable to make a decision unless all practicable steps to help them to do so have been taken without success.

3. A person is not to be treated as unable to make a decision merely because they make an unwise decision.

4. Any action taken or decision made under this act for, or on behalf of, a person who lacks capacity must be in their best interests.

Key learning point

It is important that you understand the principles of the MHA and the MCA so you can apply them in your everyday practice.

The complex nature of issues faced by offenders with mental disorders

Complex issues

It is useful to think about individuals' journeys into secure forensic settings. While common themes do arise when looking at a number of case histories – not forgetting that these themes can be useful in planning care and managing risk – it is important not to place any person in a category or box them into a defined pattern of behaviour. Detainees are individuals and must be supported as such.

5. Any action taken or decision made for, or on behalf of, a person who is deemed to lack capacity should be done so in a way that is least restrictive of their rights and freedom of action.

Practice activity

Read the following case study. How would the principles of the MHA and MCA impact on your practice in this case? You may want to make some notes.

Marlene, a 21-year-old woman, is living on your ward after being transferred from HMP Strange. She presents as a cocky young woman with a 'motormouth', and she is jumpy and overly cautious. Finding it hard to settle in the ward, Marlene uses self-harming behaviour as a way of coping. When she perceives herself to be under threat Marlene can resort to assaults, but if staff members do not intervene physically she will calm down. Marlene's mother has stated that she does not want anything to do with her anymore and the staff have noticed that Marlene is becoming more and more withdrawn, exploding more quickly at perceived slights and challenges. Marlene is very streetwise and quick-witted; she does not suffer fools and can be more than cutting in her remarks. This has made her vulnerable to assaults from others on the ward and subject to intolerance from members of the staff group.

Case study

James is a 34-year-old man with a moderate learning disability and a history of sexual offences against children. He was also abused himself over a period of 17 years by members of his family, carers and by two priests who offered him 'shelter' when he was 15 years old.

James' own offence history did not become known until one of his victims in a children's home where he was a resident ran away and informed a trusted social worker that James had abused him. The boy was nine years old and James was 15. This incident prompted James to run away and fall victim to being abused again.

James was finally arrested and charged with a number of what turned out to be increasingly serious sexual assaults. His index offence was against a six-year-old boy whom he abducted from a school playground at the age of 24. The boy was found barely alive two weeks later after being sexually assaulted and tortured.

James has been moved from a secure unit to a low secure unit in order to gain the skills he needs to be reintegrated back into wider society.

James presents as a friendly and very care-worn individual who has been victimised and treated unfairly all his life.

He has an excellent singing voice and would like to take part in The X Factor and become famous. Then he would like to live in Spain. James thinks that if he lived in Spain everything would be different and he could buy a flat and get a job. He would also like to pay society back for the trouble he has been in and work for a children's charity, but if he won The X Factor that goal would have to wait.

James becomes very weepy when his offences are mentioned and will withdraw, blaming the staff member for not understanding that that was the past and he is doing his time and attending the groups. He says, 'It is very unfair that staff keep on about it.'

James likes making staff members' drinks and toast in the morning and denies that he was caught masturbating into one of the staff member's coffees in one of his previous units.

There was a recent heated debate in James' ward round recently when two members of the clinical team criticised another member for stating that he thought James was still at risk of re-offending.

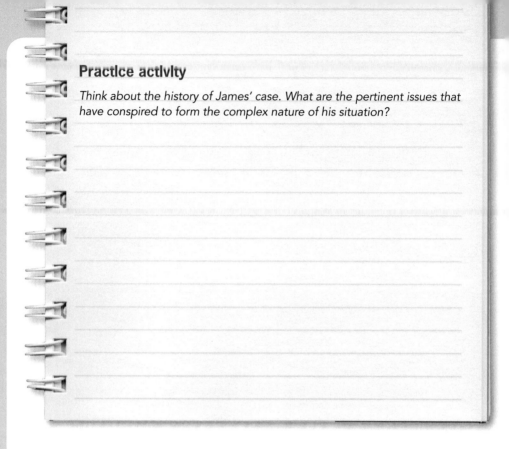

Practice activity

Think about the history of James' case. What are the pertinent issues that have conspired to form the complex nature of his situation?

A vulnerable adult and an offender

It is important to examine and acknowledge the complex nature of working with individuals who are both vulnerable adults and offenders. It is often the case that we do not view an individual as a whole person, but according to categories we have assigned to them. The notion of dialectic or trilectic issues can help us to understand how our judgement and perception can affect the care and treatment of an offender.

Dialectic and trilectic issues

Dialectic issues

To understand dialectic issues, imagine a single piece of string, knotted at each end. Both of the two knots represent ideas, philosophies, values or beliefs that are in direct opposition to each other.

For example, 'there are fairies' at one end and 'there are no fairies' at the other end – these two opposing ideas could bring conflict.

Figure 1.1: Dialectic issues

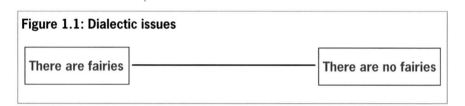

Take two, more realistic ideas:

1. Offenders with mental disorders are here because they are 'bad'.

2. Offenders with mental disorders are here because they are 'ill'.

Trilectic issues

Now imagine that with three pieces of string:

Figure 1.2: Trilectic issues

How do you negotiate a realistic workable position? How do you stop being drawn into one of the positions at the extremities of the string?

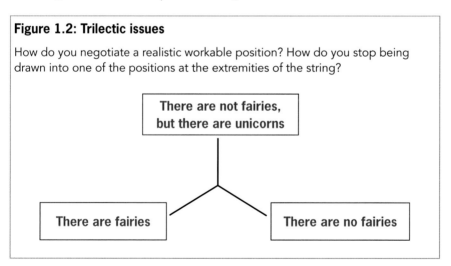

Now let's see that using the example of an offender with a mental disorder:

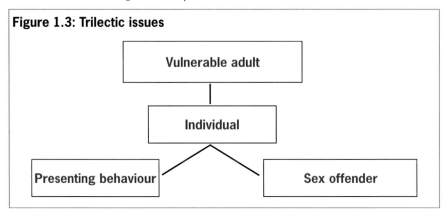

Figure 1.3: Trilectic issues

Difficulties can arise when someone is viewed not as a whole person but as one of the categories expressed at the end of one of the strings.

If a person is seen in terms of being a vulnerable adult, their presenting behaviours or a sex offender, it will have an impact on:

- the care and treatment that is being provided
- the assessment of risk
- the management of risk
- staff members' perception of the individual
- staff members' ability to work with the individual.

You may have come to some of the following conclusions when thinking about how a person is affected by us not viewing them as a whole person.

The care and treatment that is being provided: Care and treatment focused on only one aspect fails to address the holistic needs of the person. It can lead to the person being seen as the label:

'They are a victim/offender/dangerous/etc.' The individual will not progress safely and therapeutically through their journey.

The assessment of risk: Risk can either be diminished or increased depending on the perception of the risk. Taking into account only the behaviour presented on one day could bring about a failure to consider the offence behaviour, as would only seeing the person as a vulnerable adult.

Thinking activity

What are the potential risks of failing to see a person as an individual and instead seeing them in terms of their behaviours?

The management of risk: If you focus on one aspect of the offender's presentation it impacts on the management of risk. Seeing an individual only as an offender may lead to a risk averse/punitive management strategy. Seeing the person only as a vulnerable adult may lead to an overly liberal approach to risk. In seeing only the individual's presenting behaviour you fail to manage the offender with a mental disorder as a person and manage only the behaviour. This leads to a cycle of behaviour and management of behaviour. The negative impact of 'going nowhere' weighs heavily on both staff members and on the individual.

Staff members' perception of the individual: The staff member's relationship with an individual can be affected enormously by their perception of the person, not just of the offence, but also of the person's behaviour. Let's suppose that the person is sociable and polite – is there a danger of perceiving them as less of a risk because they are 'OK' or 'not that bad, really'? The answer is yes.

Staff members' individual ability to work with the offender with a mental disorder: Perception of an offender with a mental disorder can create barriers to being able to care for and treat the individual. Crimes against children and old people, or bizarre and graphic index offences can haunt the interactions between staff members and the offender.

Practice activity

Using the information you have read up to this point in the guide, reflect on your personal experiences and record the challenges you have experienced. Make sure you keep staff and patient confidentiality.

Think about:
- *the challenge of a 'demanding' individual on staff time*
- *an emotionally challenging individual who seeks to provoke a response*
- *a verbally aggressive or physically aggressive individual.*

When you have finished, you may wish to discuss the challenges you have faced with your colleagues.

The nature and purpose of a secure forensic mental health facility

The role of a secure forensic mental health facility

Individuals within secure forensic units will be detained under a section of the MHA.

The purpose of any secure forensic mental health unit can be taken from the purpose principle of the MHA Code of Practice (DH, 2008):

'Decisions under the act must be taken with a view to minimising the undesirable effects of mental disorder, by maximising the safety and well-being (mental and physical) of patients, promoting their recovery and protecting other people from harm.'

The safety and well-being of individuals and the protection of others form the basic role of secure forensic facilities. The fences, locked doors, restricted items and controlled access form part of that role. If a person is deemed to present a level of risk that would compromise their own or others' safety and they have an underlying mental disorder, then a secure forensic facility is an option for managing that risk.

Secure units

There are different levels of security depending on the level of danger and the immediacy of the risk presented. Those individuals who display a high level of dangerous behaviour and who are likely to present an immediate risk

may end up in either high or medium secure hospitals depending on the nature of the danger and the potential consequences of the risk.

As the likelihood of the danger decreases, and in line with the MHA Code of Practice least restrictive principle (DH, 2008), the necessity for the higher level of security decreases. Other secure forensic facilities include low secure and locked rehabilitation.

There are approximately 4,500 places in high and medium secure services, with around 800 in high secure facilities. In July 2007 88% were male and 12% female (DH, 2008). Around 84% were aged 26–64, although since that time there has been an increase in females aged 18–26 due to the amendments to the MHA in 2007.

A myth about security

There is a myth within secure services that the level of risk diminishes as offenders move through the levels of security. The gravity may change due to the environmental inhibitors; however, the underlying risk may still exist. For example, a child offender in a high secure unit should have little opportunity to re-offend due to the nature of the security that maintains public safety. However, as the person moves through levels to medium and then low security units, the opportunities to offend increase. There is less restriction on access to local communities through increased leave. Whilst this is a therapeutic necessity to enable recovery and reintegration, it is imperative that there is no complacency in the approach to security and the management of risk.

Restricted patients

There are a number of individuals that are not only detained under the MHA but who also have restrictions imposed upon them by the Ministry of Justice. This group of offenders with mental disorders, while protected under the MHA, are subject to Ministry of Justice approval for major changes in their care and management and cannot be discharged without their authority.

The role of secure forensic facilities

As stated in the introduction, the purpose of secure forensic services is to keep the individual and the public safe and to provide appropriate treatment in order to mitigate harm. This may on occasion, due to the chronic nature and degree of risk, include the provision of care to a small number of individuals who present a long-term risk to society.

Thinking activity

As a result of your reading, has your view of the purpose of secure forensic mental health services changed?

The history of secure forensic facilities, then and now

The origins of secure forensic facilities

'Madhouses' have been around since the 1700s, when many were no more than utility services providing 'asylum' for the unwanted, wretched and unfortunate. Many, such as Bedlam in London (which was first founded in 1247), became places of amusement for those who could afford a penny to look around.

By the mid-18th century a new philanthropy was creeping into society and the science of the mind was becoming fashionable. With it came the political change that saw the first secure hospital, Broadmoor, open in 1863.

Broadmoor was now a place for the criminally insane, the dangerous lunatic and the mad murderer. It was a place of both incarceration and with the growing 'science' of psychiatry, a place to treat the offender. There were few treatment options available apart from social psychiatry; however, with the coming of drug-based and physical treatments this changed rapidly.

Over the coming years Rampton and Ashworth Hospitals followed. Along with Broadmoor, these high secure hospitals were self-sufficient, having workshops, kitchens and other functions carried out by the patients. Ward staff were not trained in any specific way and functioned under a physician superintendent.

The 20th century

At the beginning of the 20th century, Rampton, for example, had around 1,500 patients, with individuals being detained there for many years.

There were many people detained within secure facilities who should never have been there: people with learning disabilities, children who were a 'nuisance' and patients with a mental illness for which, at that time, there was no treatment. The high secure hospitals would then work with the large psychiatric hospitals if any individual was deemed safe enough to move on.

This system worked without any major change until the 1960s when the then Health Minister Enoch Powell campaigned for the closure of the large psychiatric hospitals, which began to happen in the mid-1970s under the banner of 'care in the community'. By coincidence, there was a major inquiry into Rampton Hospital at around the same time, which brought high secure hospitals into the spotlight.

These two developments brought about the changes that helped to shape today's secure forensic services. The high secure hospitals were under scrutiny and it was found that they were housing individuals who did not need to be in high secure units. The relationship between the high secure hospitals and the large psychiatric hospitals no longer existed, so where could the people who needed to move on be moved on to? The answer lay in the establishment of medium secure services, smaller units (not asylum sized) that would provide safe care and treatment.

Present day services

The closure of the large psychiatric hospitals resulted in an increase in people with mental health problems in the prison services, the majority of whom did not need high secure care. This created a service gap and from the 1980s private healthcare providers have been seeking to provide the necessary beds funded by the NHS. There are now many private healthcare providers running medium, low and locked rehabilitation facilities, all under the auspices of the Care Quality Commission (as are NHS facilities). There is also a growing number of NHS providers establishing secure care facilities. Over the coming years this will present a challenge to those in the private sector. Cost factors will mean that offenders with mental disorders are moved back into the NHS, leaving some in the private sector with no choice but to cease provision. There have certainly been improvements from the old 'madhouses'; staff are now trained, premises regulated and laws passed to protect the rights of

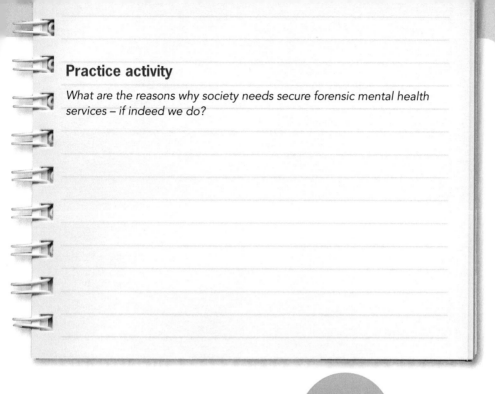

Practice activity

What are the reasons why society needs secure forensic mental health services – if indeed we do?

the people being detained. However, what remains at the heart of any service 'then or now' is the humanity with which the care is being delivered (DH, 2012).

Keeping people safe

In the foreword to the Mental Health Act Code of Practice (DH, 2008), Alan Johnson stated: 'It is important that we have a modern legal framework within which clinicians can intervene where necessary to protect people with mental disorders themselves and, sometimes, to protect other people as well. But with the power to intervene comes the responsibility to do so only where it is right and to the highest standards possible.'

Thinking activity

How do secure forensic facilities keep people safe? Who are the people we have a duty of care to keep safe?

From this statement we can take it that more than one area of safety is covered:

1. That a person's detention is legally 'safe' under the law.

2. That the rights of the individual who is detained are safe under the law and in practice.

3. That the person being detained is kept safe, mentally and physically.
4. That the public are kept safe from the potential consequences of a detained person's behaviour.
5. That the practice that is being delivered to the patient group is safe.
6. That the staff who work within such facilities are safe.

Safety is the underlying premise of secure forensic care.

Therapy vs. security

There is a very interesting (dialectic) tension between therapy and security.

While this tension exists people working within secure settings will have problems in their delivery of care. Staff members who take a therapy-based approach may be seen as being 'weak' – too soft in their approach, while those who fall on the side of security may be seen as 'hard' – too punitive in their approach. The nature of the care provided by a service will be dependent on the views of the stronger more influential voice. This can also lead to care swinging between having a therapeutic or security focus, depending on which voice is louder at any one particular time. Imagine how this must make the person feel.

There is no practical way of changing the dialectic, as neither end is correct on its own: therapy cannot override security and security cannot undermine therapy. A new model must be created to demonstrate not the therapy versus security model, but how therapy sits within a secure setting:

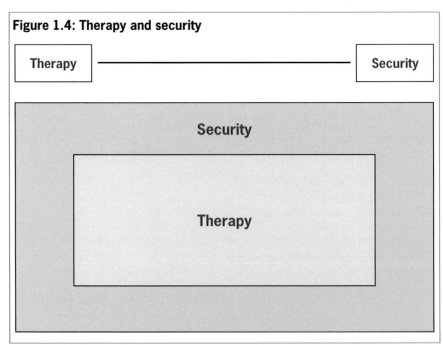

Figure 1.4: Therapy and security

Therapy ——————————————— Security

Security

Therapy

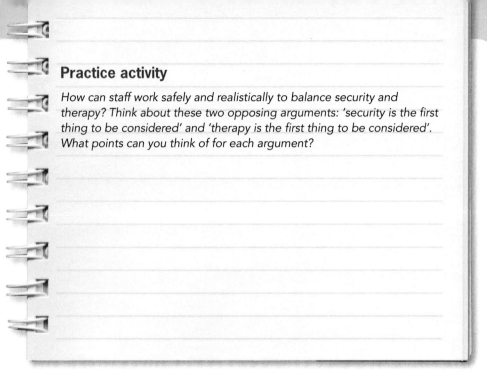

Therapy needs to be delivered within the framework of high-quality physical, procedural and relational security (DH, 2010). Within security there must be flexibility to enable therapeutic risk taking and recovery.

The only time when security must take precedent is when there is the potential for a major incident, or when such an incident has occurred. Even so, this should be for the shortest possible time, to the least restrictive principle, carried out with respect and taking into consideration the dignity of the individual/s involved.

Security should not be used as an excuse to punitively impinge on an individual's rights.

In thinking about security vs. therapy, services should seek to deliver therapy in a safe and secure way. This will create an alliance between the two factors.

Person-centredness, empowerment, advocacy and active participation in the care of offenders with mental disorders

Understand patient participation

According to the MHA Code of Practice (DH, 2008) patient participation is one of the five principles on which the whole of the MHA stands. This in turn demonstrates the principles by which we must practise in our delivery of care.

The participation principle states that: *'Patients must be given the opportunity to be involved, as far as is practicable in the circumstances, in planning, developing and reviewing their own treatment and care to help ensure that it is delivered in a way that is as appropriate and effective as possible.'*

This sentence leaves no doubt that the person must be empowered to take part in, as far as is practicable, every aspect of their care. In order for individuals to be able to participate, they need:

- correct information
- appropriate support through the provision of:
  - advocacy
  - education
  - emotional support
  - safe management strategies
  - meaningful assessment
  - realistic goals
  - practical support
  - equal opportunities
  - access.

This may also include taking into consideration any advance wishes or statements made by the person for any occasions when they are unable to participate in their care owing to increased symptomology, changes in behavioural risk factors, negative impact of social changes etc. Advance wishes and statements should be documented and act as a point of referral when formulating care, treatment and risk management plans.

Enabling individuals to participate in their care and treatment is a powerful tool in building meaningful relationships with them as it demonstrates respect.

The activity of patient participation should be documented clearly in the

person's clinical records, supported with statements such as:

- 'in conversation with...'
- 'when ... and I talked about...'
- 'in reviewing ... care plans we...'
- 'when ... spoke with me about...'

These statements evidence meaningful interactions between staff and individuals in their care. Risk issues can impact on an individual's ability to access opportunities and activities. In these cases participation must focus on reducing the risk and getting the individual to a point where they are able to do so.

The advantages of individuals being involved in their own care could include:

- the person feeling included and therefore being less challenging of their care and treatment
- the person feeling more empowered and therefore being more willing to engage in their care
- shortening the period that the individual needs to be detained
- the reduction of risk behaviour.

Therapeutic use of self

The definitions of 'therapeutic use of self' include:

1. *'The total essence or being of a person; the individual'*
2. *'Those affective, cognitive, and spiritual qualities that distinguish one person from another; individuality'*
3. *'A person's awareness of his or her own being or identity; consciousness; ego'*

(*Mosby's Medical Dictionary*, 2009)

In order to use yourself in a therapeutic way you must understand that self-awareness is the key to doing so successfully.

Working with often difficult, complex and challenging individuals can stir up feelings within staff that can have a detrimental effect on them, their ability to work effectively, and their relationships with the people they support, and colleagues. It can also impact on their life and relationships outside of work. While the individual member of staff may be aware that something is not quite right, they may not be aware of the cause of the issue, or of the impact it is having upon them or others. This can leave the member of staff vulnerable and at risk.

Individuals can only work effectively when they are managing themselves, their interactions with the patient group and communication with their colleagues. It is very difficult to manage yourself without an awareness of what is going on around you emotionally, physically and socially.

The use of colleagues to give feedback, supervision, training

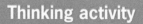

Thinking activity

How can you support individuals to take part in their own care?

and appraisal is an essential factor in gaining self-awareness and the awareness of how interactions with offenders and colleagues are developing. Many individuals shy away from gaining feedback, either out of a false sense of how well they are doing or out of fear that they will be 'told off' or criticised.

The people we support may also 'press buttons' to test out if we do 'what we say on the tin' or if we resort to impatient, unfriendly or other negative intervention styles. In this way, the people we support can be the best 'teachers' of performance if they are allowed to be.

Staff interventions will have either a positive or negative impact. Admittedly, the majority of communications with offenders with mental disorders have low-risk impacts and the results do not dramatically increase or decrease the level of risk. However, if we are not aware of what the impact of that intervention may be, or if we ignore what it tells us, then the risk may increase quickly, resulting in a dangerous situation. By demonstrating in practice the therapeutic use of self, we can reduce risk, build and maintain meaningful relationships, and promote patient recovery.

It is integral that staff working in secure forensic facilities are aware that the way they work with offenders with mental disorders is an essential part of the individual's care, treatment and recovery.

Building meaningful relationships

While it is wrong to have anything other than a professional relationship

with an individual you are supporting, that relationship needs to be therapeutic. That doesn't mean a relationship that is based on therapy; it means a relationship that is genuine and meaningful. This depends on the way in which we engage with the people we support in our day-to-day interactions with them.

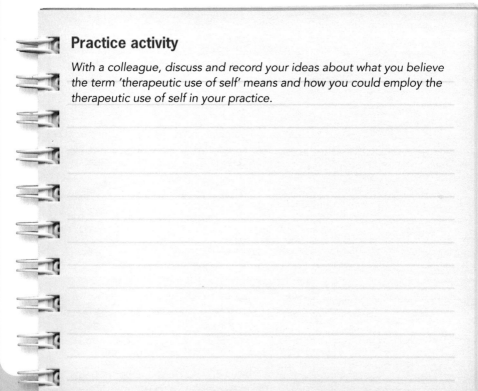

Practice activity

With a colleague, discuss and record your ideas about what you believe the term 'therapeutic use of self' means and how you could employ the therapeutic use of self in your practice.

The individuals we care for spend a lot of time watching us and gaining an understanding of how we engage with the people around us. That includes other offenders, colleagues, professionals and visitors. They build a profile of the people they feel that they can trust. This of course includes how you relate to them too.

Individuals will judge our actions. For example, they may be looking to see whether we are:

- honest
- reliable
- trustworthy
- fair
- loud
- cynical
- hard
- soft
- understanding
- knowledgeable
- lazy
- bullying
- always 'right'.

We can begin to build a meaningful relationship by ensuring that the intention behind our actions is based upon a genuine interest in the individual's welfare. People will pick up, just by the way that we interact, if we don't seem to care, or if we seem bored or angry.

Imagine you want to have a serious conversation with someone about an

Thinking activity

What risks do you think can arise when staff members are not 'fair' across the group of people they support?

important issue. However, when you try to talk to the person you receive a disinterested, 'couldn't care less' response. How would you feel?

When working with individuals in your care, you need to cultivate and build an open, genuine and meaningful relationship.

In order to build a good relationship with someone, you will need to display the following key attributes:

- honesty
- reliability
- trust
- capability (being good at your job)
- fairness
- being proactive
- humour (laughing with not at people we are supporting, and being able to laugh at yourself)
- active listening.

Therapeutic boundaries

How do you maintain therapeutic boundaries?

Therapeutic boundaries are clear and sensible demarcations that ensure a safer relationship between staff and the individuals they support.

Thinking activity

What do you understand about the term 'therapeutic boundaries'?

Figure 1.5: Therapeutic boundaries

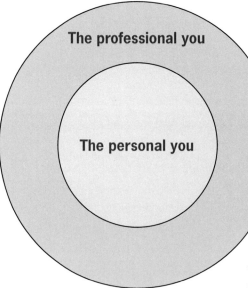

Boundaries can be defined as:

- the external boundaries between you and the individual you are supporting
  - the internal boundary between the 'personal you' and the 'professional' you.

The external boundaries relate to the physical and personal space between us and the individual. Do we encroach too much into it? Do we avoid it? Do we ignore it? Encroaching into it or avoiding it can have catastrophic consequences. Boundaries need to be negotiated with the person and within the policies and practice of where you work.

The internal boundaries relate to the distinction between the 'personal' you and the 'professional' you. In your professional role you must be yourself but the individuals you support do not need you to be their friend; trying to be their friend will not build a better therapeutic relationship.

What are the boundaries?

One of the most common difficulties encountered by staff working within secure forensic facilities is that of maintaining therapeutic boundaries.

Offenders with mental disorders respond to clear, uncomplicated boundaries that enable them to feel emotionally safe and therapeutically secure. Lack of clarity and complicated boundaries will leave them feeling unsafe and insecure and will lead to increased risk behaviours and leave staff members vulnerable to assault and/or allegations.

Thinking activity

Can you think of any more subjects that it would be inappropriate to discuss with individuals in your care?

What is it appropriate to talk about?

Personal information should be kept to a minimum and should stay within the guidelines set by the service where you work. There are some clear nos. Do not discuss:

- where you live
- details of personal relationships
- family dynamics
- your sex life
- advice on personal issues based on your own experience
- your nights out
- your own personal history.

Instead, you need to reflect upon information that you are allowed and is safe to share. Examples could include:

- hobbies
- musical taste
- soaps
- news items
- fashion
- films
- books.

In order to build a meaningful relationship and maintain therapeutic boundaries, each of us has to develop a sense of who we are professionally whilst still being ourselves within the role we undertake.

Most of the time boundaries are subject to 'slippage' – odd lapses in awareness, or moments of tiredness, boredom, complacency or over-familiarity. Sometimes boundaries are crossed due to a member of staff thinking they know better, over-confidence, fear, not knowing the risks or underestimating the risks.

Sadly, boundaries can be violated; this happens when a person knowingly and intentionally breaks through the boundary. This is abuse of the relationship.

The challenges to maintaining therapeutic boundaries in practice could include:

- over-familiarity
- fear
- ignorance

- complacency
- knowing better than the offender
- boredom
- over-confidence
- underestimating the risk involved.

How views and attitudes impact on the lives of offenders with mental disorders and their families

Thinking activity

How can you stop people being labelled within your ward/unit?

The impact of labelling individuals

Labelling within secure forensic mental health services only concretes divisions, creating a culture that sees 'them and us', 'haves and have nots', 'included and excluded', 'treatables and untreatables', 'timewasters and wastes of time'.

Practice activity

What impact could negative labels have on:
- *a person's family*
- *an offender*
- *staff members working with offenders with mental illnesses.*

People may be labelled as: a person with schizophrenia; parent of a person with schizophrenia; person with depression; journalist; priest; politician; person with Down's syndrome; person who self-harms; teacher; burglar.

Offenders can also label staff members too. Are you or your colleagues aware of any labels you may wear within your workplace?

Thinking activity

How would you feel if someone was demonstrating a negative behaviour?

Promoting positive attitudes

There is a need to promote positive attitudes to mental illness within the workplace and wider society. For example:

- individuals with mental illness can be and are active members of society
- only very few people diagnosed with mental illnesses commit offences, serious or otherwise
- mental illness can affect anyone.

The media and offenders with mental disorders

The media often has a negative influence on people's perceptions of offenders with mental disorders. Very often, offenders with mental disorders are labelled as 'nutters', 'schizos', 'psychos', 'manipulative' and 'time wasters'. How might these labels and those that the media uses impact on you – how and where you work?

Promoting positive communication with offenders who have mental disorders

Negative styles of communication

Negative forms of communication can include being disinterested (yawning, looking at your watch or glancing at the door), aggressive (stern facial gestures and hand movements), overbearing (intruding in someone's personal space, standing over someone when they are seated), passive (poor eye contact, defensive body language).

Positive communication

Communication has three main components:

1. Content – 7%
2. Intonation (tone of voice) – 23%
3. Non-verbal (body language) – 70%

Evolutionary psychology means that we are hardwired to observe all three elements of communication in our interactions with other people. We automatically check the three components to see if they match. For example, a person can say they are interested in what you are saying, but if their eyes wander to the clock and their tone of voice suggests that they can't really be bothered, you are unlikely to believe them. Imagine how that would make you feel if you were a patient and you had something important to say?

In our everyday interactions with the individuals we support we have to be very aware of our communication.

Sometimes we have to provide support to our patients, challenge their behaviour, guide them, share difficult news or have a laugh. It is important that we do not become complacent in the way that we communicate, or dismiss or trivialise their issues. The people we support are restricted,

locked up in an environment that they may feel is 'unsafe' or 'uncaring' and what may seem to be a very small issue to us can become a big issue for the individuals we are supporting. Our communication needs to demonstrate an attitude of understanding.

We also need to be aware of what it is about the person we are communicating with that can make us negative in our communication. If we are not aware of this then it will impact negatively on the relationship. Negative communication can also increase the risk of self-harming behaviour or harm to others.

If someone feels badly about themselves and you demonstrate dismissive communication, you can 'concrete' in the person's mind that they must be bad for you to dismiss them.

Positive communication will promote a therapeutic relationship and will bring about a level of trust that is very important to support recovery.

Thinking activity

What are the benefits of positive communication?

Positive communication must also be maintained, as it can easily be lost, even through a one-off remark.

Just as with the patient group, we must ensure that we provide positive communication with an individual's relatives, carers and friends to help maintain their social network and support system.

Thinking activity

Think about the function of reflective practice within your role. Have you found your experience of supervision and reflective practice useful?

Using reflective practice to check the effectiveness of communication

Reflective practice

Reflective practice provides a space where two or more members of staff can safely explore and discuss issues that can affect the quality of care delivered to their patient group and their relationships with individuals, relatives, carers or friends. It is based on openness.

Reflective practice requires:

- honesty
- focus
- trust
- openness
- willingness to listen
- willingness to challenge
- willingness to be challenged.

Reflective practice is normally carried out with someone who is an experienced facilitator who can demonstrate confidence and competence. It can either be formal or informal in nature.

Reflective practice needs a basic structure, even if that is just a beginning, a middle and an end.

1. The beginning is the subject, which may be decided after an incident or an intervention.

2. The middle is the discussion, which may ask some of the following questions.
   - What do you feel?
   - What do you think?
   - What went well?
   - What could be improved upon?

3. The end is the action planning – 'how do we move things forward?'

Reflective practice is not a chance to moan or a place to be told off, nor is it part of the appraisal process. It is a tool for checking what you are doing, to explain and examine how things are going for you, and to stop negative issues building up that could impact on the care you deliver.

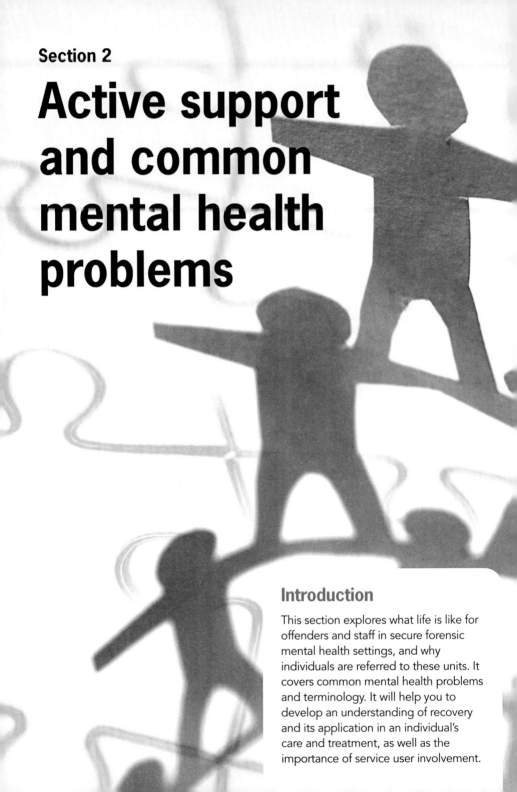

Active support and common mental health problems

Introduction

This section explores what life is like for offenders and staff in secure forensic mental health settings, and why individuals are referred to these units. It covers common mental health problems and terminology. It will help you to develop an understanding of recovery and its application in an individual's care and treatment, as well as the importance of service user involvement.

The provision of active support for individuals detained in secure forensic mental health settings is essential. Active support has a meaningful purpose, which minimises the undesirable effects of mental disorders by maximising the safety and well-being (mental and physical) of individuals, promoting their recovery and protecting other people from harm. It demonstrates respect and encourages the participation of the individual and seeks to maintain the therapeutic relationship and support therapeutic boundaries. It also seeks to minimise the negative effects of boredom, isolation and frustration that living in a secure environment can cause.

How active support translates into person-centred interventions

What is life like for individuals and staff in secure forensic mental health settings?

No matter what our circumstances are, there are activities that make our lives enjoyable and productive, for example, going out with friends, family outings, reading a book or watching a film. Another important factor is having the freedom to pursue and have relationships and to experience intimacy. Individuals in secure forensic settings often do not have these freedoms.

Patients in secure forensic settings sometimes report feeling:

Thinking activity

How would you feel if the things that make your life enjoyable were taken away and you were 'locked up' in a secure environment with people you did not know?

- isolated
- frustrated
- angry
- disempowered
- lonely
- in the dark
- unsafe
- invisible
- forgotten
- suicidal
- sexually frustrated
- like cattle
- without hope.

It is important to keep these feelings in mind as you interact with the individuals in your care. You can go home at the end of your shift and do the things you want to, but offenders cannot.

The potential impact on staff

Working with a challenging group of offenders with mental disorders, with their own histories and tragedies, living in what can be a hostile environment, can impact on staff physically, emotionally and intellectually.

Staff members have reported feelings of:

- frustration
- irritability
- impatience
- fear
- disempowerment
- isolation
- being uninformed
- being unsupported
- being 'in the dark'.

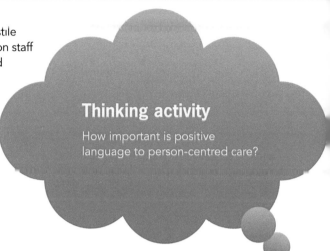

Thinking activity

How important is positive language to person-centred care?

The organisational politics of services and the behaviour of the detainees can all have an impact on staff.

You need to ensure that the things you share about yourself will not make you vulnerable, and that you maintain therapeutic boundaries and use yourself therapeutically. Clinical supervision and reflective practice can support staff in maintaining a high level of professionalism and active support.

Factors that could decrease the negative impacts on staff could include:

- access to clinical supervision and reflective practice
- training to support interactions with offenders with mental disorders
- working in a non-defensive environment.

Isolation or a lack of help and support could increase negative impacts on staff members.

The impact of language and terminology in secure forensic mental health settings

Staff can find that they start using language and terminology that describes the offenders they are working with in negative or pejorative ways. They may have heard the language or terms used in the media or by others they are working with. For example, as covered in Section 1, offenders with mental health problems are often called 'troublemakers', 'self-harmers', 'manipulators' or 'personality disordered'. Staff may find that they begin their sentences with 'He's doing my head in…', 'If she does that again…', 'If you keep on doing that, you won't get anything…' and 'You are really winding me up'. These terms and phrases are unhelpful and can be counterproductive when working with people in a person-centred way.

Inclusive language must be used in documentation to record the involvement of the individual within their care. For example, 'We talked about...'

The language culture needs to move away from using words with negative connotations, for example, using the word 'cutlery' instead of the word 'sharps'.

Staff need to be aware of the potential negative impact of defining an offender with a mental disorder by their diagnosis or behaviour.

Recovery in secure forensic mental health settings

The basics of recovery

The underlying principle of recovery is empowerment, but within a secure forensic facility the environment can make the implementation of the recovery model challenging – it is hard for individuals to feel empowered when their movement and activities are being controlled.

Factors that influence recovery include:

- a stable living environment
- opportunities for personal growth
- financial stability
- freedom of expression of cultural and spiritual beliefs
- freedom of expression of sexuality
- the development of 'good' relationships
- a sense of belonging
- a sense of control over their life.

> **Key learning point**
>
> The offender is a person, not a description or a diagnosis.

These recovery factors are underpinned by:

- seeing the person as a whole and not just their 'symptoms' or behaviour
- understanding that people can change and recover
- emphasising that recovery is a journey rather than a final destination
- a flexible and individualised approach
- hope.

It can be difficult for individuals to have hope when they are in a restricted environment. This could be because of their past history, or feelings of disempowerment, anger or loneliness. However, there are factors that can promote recovery even in the most challenging of environments.

For example, many of the individuals we support have low self-esteem, self-worth and self-belief. Where this is the case, we need to demonstrate a belief that they can change and that they have the ability to do so. Listening to individuals actively and genuinely also helps. However, listening without action can be empty. Actions demonstrate our understanding.

Individuals need to have access to the relevant information and explanations for things that impact on their lives. When an individual has lost hope, staff need to promote hopefulness and encourage them to believe that things can change and that they can get through situations. Realistic expectations and goals are needed. Enabling the individual to be included in their care and treatment will support their recovery.

Thinking activity

How can you facilitate an offender's recovery?

Understanding user involvement

What is the difference between patient participation and user involvement?

Patient participation is a person's involvement in their own care, treatment, decision-making and personal development. It is an important factor in their recovery, an enabling function and part of the therapeutic process.

User involvement provides the opportunity for individuals to be involved in the running, development and decision-making processes of a ward, unit or organisation. User involvement is not a box-ticking exercise but the meaningful involvement of people in forums that promote positive change.

Patient participation is a vital factor in the care and treatment of all offenders with mental disorders and should be enabled and encouraged at all times. It is personal and fundamental to their recovery. User involvement is also important, however, it is less concerned with an individual's personal care and treatment than with the opportunities for influence and involvement in their environment.

There is a link between patient participation and user involvement, as lack of appropriate support to be actively involved in user forums can impact negatively on individuals' mental health and hinder their ability to participate positively in their own care. Positive involvement in user forums will benefit their mental health and promote their participation in their own care and treatment.

Organisations should have forums for patient involvement, for example:

- community meetings
- patient or service user councils
- activity planning meetings

- daily planning meetings
- food groups
- recruitment activity
- marketing and service promotion
- network groups and forums
- conferences.

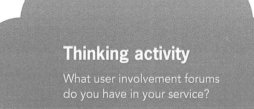

Thinking activity

What user involvement forums do you have in your service?

It is important to realise that user involvement is not solely about individuals attending these forums; they must be able to actively participate in them. This may mean that some preparation work has to be done prior to their attendance. It also means that relevant information must be available in an appropriate format.

Some individuals may need assistance to attend user involvement activities, which may mean that staff, family members, advocates or volunteers provide support. User forums should be welcoming and non-patronising. They should take into account the needs of the group and be flexible to accommodate them. For example,

for a group of individuals with poor concentration skills it would be wrong to schedule a long meeting with a lengthy agenda and reams of minutes.

Organisations can learn a lot from the people in their care if they give them a voice and genuinely listen.

The circumstances and problems that can lead individuals to secure forensic mental health services

Where are individuals referred from and how do they arrive in a secure forensic mental health setting?

Individuals arrive in secure forensic mental health settings from a number of places and for a number of reasons. Individuals may arrive via:

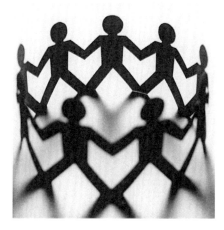

- court, for either assessment or for treatment and care
- prison
- admission from non-secure facilities
- admission from a higher level of security as part of their treatment pathway
- admission from a lower level of security due to an increase in risky behaviour
- transfer across from the same level of security as part of their treatment pathway, to be nearer their home, for example another unit:
  - for a specific treatment approach
  - due to a commissioning decision based on a clinical or financial need
  - in response to a safeguarding issue, for example, individuals were transferred from Winterbourne View in 2011 due to the ill treatment of the people there.

Depending on their personal circumstances, individuals will respond differently to their admission or transfer. No matter what the reasons for their arrival, individuals will have a level of anxiety about the change that can impact on their transition into their new environment. We should be aware of this and ensure that we manage this transition sensitively and safely. Remember that a number of offenders who are admitted have had a vast experience of being 'in care' – not all of it positive; so every effort should be made to build up trust and establish

a therapeutic relationship. Some individuals know the 'system' better than the staff who care for them, so it is important to observe and assess risk following their arrival. Remember that all individuals will be sectioned under the MHA.

Common mental health problems

Obsessive compulsive disorder (OCD)

Obsessions are unwelcome and intrusive thoughts that can create ideas and impulses that recur within the mind, for example, thinking 'My hands are dirty, my hands are dirty,' followed by the compulsion to carry out the act of washing the hands. The more intrusive and pervading the thought, and the more compelled the individual is to act upon the thought, the greater the problem. Many people live with and find ways to manage their OCD.

Anxiety disorder

Anxiety disorder is characterised by constant worry over what can be very ordinary and everyday things. The unrealistic worries that lead to anxiety can result in physical symptoms such as restlessness, sleeplessness, weight loss, palpitations, headaches and indigestion, and psychological problems such as panic attacks, eating disorders or OCD.

Depression

Depression is like a huge cloud settling upon a person, bringing with it a lowering of mood, feelings of guilt, hopelessness or worthlessness, and a sense of failure and doom. Depression can also trigger suicidal thoughts. It can affect relationships, work and social life, which in turn can bring feelings of isolation and loneliness. Depression can range from being mild to being very severe. It is often linked to anxiety.

Schizophrenia

Schizophrenia is very misunderstood 'disease' and can be seen more as a collection of symptoms rather than an actual illness. People can experience a vast range of symptoms to varying degrees.

Symptoms can include:

- delusions ie. false beliefs and ideas
- confusion
- withdrawal – social and emotional
- depression
- loss of contact with reality
- loss of motivation
- hallucinations (false perceptions), which can include:
  - hearing noises that aren't there (including voices)
  - seeing things that aren't there
  - feelings of being touched
  - smelling strange odours.

Eating disorders

Individuals with eating disorders have an obsession with their eating habits and are also likely to have a very poor body image. Eating disorders are often linked with anxiety and can have elements of OCD. Eating disorder can involve the urge to lose or to gain weight.

Factors that can affect mental health

It is important to remember that it is generally a number of factors that have brought individuals into services and it can be difficult to know which precipitated their admission. Any problem that affects an individual's mental health could be a factor in their admission.

Some things to consider

Different people will respond differently to the same situations; this is down to their individual personality and ways of coping with life.

Mental health problems can be masked by an individual's behaviour/attitude. Depression, for example, can be put down to lack of motivation or an unwillingness to engage, especially if the person has been diagnosed with a personality disorder. Individuals with a learning disability can also have mental health problems; these can be missed, especially if the person has poor communication/language skills.

Mental health problems can be triqgered by internal or external factors. Someone may watch something on the TV that triggers a 'flashback' to an earlier event in their lives. Some individuals experience auditory, visual or tactile responses to flashbacks that can be extremely distressing and cause changes in behaviour.

Individuals with a psychotic illness such as schizophrenia are very vulnerable to stress and anxiety which will exacerbate their symptoms. It will also impact on

Key learning point

You can find out further information about mental health conditions at www.mind.org.uk.

their ability to process information and respond in a rational way. Mental illness should not be used as an excuse for challenging behaviour; it should however, be taken into consideration in the planning and implementation of treatment and care.

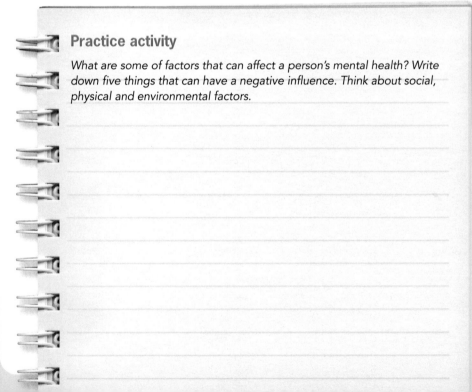

Practice activity

What are some of factors that can affect a person's mental health? Write down five things that can have a negative influence. Think about social, physical and environmental factors.

The term 'personality disorder'

The problem with the personality disorder diagnosis

Personality disorder is one of the least understood and most misrepresented terms within the overarching descriptor of mental disorder.

It could be said that everybody has a 'personality disorder' but that the majority have developed a sophisticated and socially acceptable way of interacting with their environment, have a good level of social and self-awareness and can manage their vulnerabilities. They also have the ability to change and be flexible, using their life experience to help them adapt.

However, even the most laid back of people can lose the ability to cope in a socially acceptable and responsible way. As our level of stress increases, our ability to deal with those stresses is impaired. This can cause, for example, illness, alcohol abuse, lack of sleep, at which point we can regress to less sophisticated behaviour. This alone, however, does not fit the diagnosis of personality disorder.

So what is personality disorder?

The diagnosis of personality disorder applies when a person finds it hard to cope in society – with its systems and the everyday interactions with individuals and groups. When the person can 'cope', they have a limited range of ways of doing so. They often find change difficult and have limited skills for being flexible around people and systems. This can create friction between the individual and others, and this friction can lead to clashes with social systems. For example, in school the person may be seen as disruptive, which can lead to exclusion.

Personality disorder can be socially isolating and individuals with a personality disorder have described their lives as solitary and lonely; they may feel as though they are on life's periphery. As a result, they tend to be self-reliant, angry and less likely to follow socially acceptable patterns of behaviour. They may avoid or be unable to sustain positive relationships. They may exhibit offending behaviour, including crimes of acquisition, assault, drug or alcohol offences and other antisocial behaviours.

These difficulties can also be internalised and seen in self-harming and/or suicidal behaviour. Not all people in secure units with the diagnosis of personality disorder have committed offences.

Sub-types

There are different sub-types of personality disorder, arranged into three 'clusters'.

- Cluster A: suspicious:
  - paranoid
  - schizoid
  - schizotypal
  - antisocial
- Cluster B: emotional and impulsive:
  - borderline
  - histrionic
  - narcissistic

- Cluster C: anxious:
  - avoidant
  - dependent
  - obsessive-compulsive

Causes

There are three main causational factors.

1. **Genetics:** Aspects of personality are inherited. Vulnerabilities to stress can be inherent and can be triggered by emotional distress, physical illness and/or trauma.

2. **Trauma:** Individuals who are subjected to emotional abuse and neglect, or physical and/or sexual violence on a regular basis can develop maladaptive coping mechanisms to deal with their situation.

3. **Poor, chaotic and dysfunctional upbringing:** We all need to be brought up in a safe and supportive environment in order to gain the necessary life and pro-social skills to 'navigate' our way through life and to deal with situations. Individuals with the diagnosis of personality disorder may not have that experience.

It is not generally a single factor behind an individual's diagnosis of personality disorder, but a combination.

Treatment

Treatments can include:
- cognitive behavioural therapy
- dialectical behaviour therapy
- therapeutic communities
- art and other creative therapies
- talking therapies
- medication.

The term 'mental disorder'

According to the Mental Health Act Code of Practice (DH, 2008) the term 'mental disorder' is defined as: 'any disorder or disability of the mind'. It goes on to say: 'Relevant professionals should determine whether a patient has a disorder or disability of the mind, in accordance with good clinical practice and accepted standards of what constitutes such a disorder or disability' (DH, 2008).

From a very simple perspective this could mean 'anything', as there are no clear definitions of mental health against which to judge mental disorder. This leaves the term mental disorder open to subjective interpretation, and one which is influenced by cultural and social values and beliefs. This means that individuals who are seen by 'relevant professionals' are in the hands of a system that relies

Thinking activity

How do you think the media represents people with the label of personality disorder?

on those responsible for providing 'good clinical practice and acceptable standards' (DH, 2008).

Good clinical practitioners will use accepted standards in order to make a diagnosis, which will determine the treatment pathway. They will look for significant psychopathology, the presence of signs and symptoms and also the presence of suffering. (Although not everybody with a 'mental disorder' suffers!) Treatment will therefore seek to reduce the signs and symptoms and to reduce the presence of suffering.

The only exception to the rule is: 'Dependence on drugs and alcohol is not considered to be a disorder or disability of the mind' (DH, 2008).

Learning disability is not an exception but it has additional criteria: 'A person with learning disability shall not be considered by reason of that disability to be suffering from a mental disorder… unless that disability is associated with abnormally aggressive or seriously irresponsible behaviour' (DH, 2008).

Presence of a mental disorder is a necessary requirement in order for someone to be detained under the MHA.

The term 'challenging behaviour'

The most accepted and widely used definition of challenging behaviour is: 'culturally abnormal behaviour of such intensity, frequency or duration that

Thinking activity

What influence could the label 'mentally disordered' have on an individual's reintegration into society?

the physical safety of the person or others is likely to be placed in serious jeopardy, or behaviour which is likely to seriously limit use of, or result in the person being denied access to ordinary community facilities' (Emerson, 1995).

Challenging behaviour does not occur 'out of the blue', there will be underlying causational factors such as:

- mental illness eg. anxiety, psychosis
- emotional stress eg. relationship breakdown
- environmental factors eg. ward dynamics
- change eg. new admission, a staff member leaving, transfer
- communication difficulties eg. poor vocabulary
- physical eg. pain, migraine, cold
- psychological eg. post-traumatic stress disorder (PTSD), loss, flashbacks developmental disorders eg. Asperger's syndrome, autism

- organic eg. dementia, Korsakoff's syndrome, Othello syndrome
- fear (real or perceived) eg. feeling unsafe and insecure.

It is imperative that the term 'challenging behaviour' is used in context, and that a holistic approach is used in the care and treatment of individuals who display such behaviour. An individual's treatment and care should not be centred around the challenging behaviour, as they will become defined by that behaviour rather than as a person.

The presence of challenging behaviour can lead to a diminished quality of life and exclusion from everyday aspects of society and its opportunities.

Challenging behaviour can result in:

- exclusion from local services, such as schools and healthcare
- detention
- inhibited life opportunities eg. in work, travel, relationships, education.

The service response to challenging behaviour may be:

- locked doors
- physical restraint
- seclusion.

This could include over-prescribing drugs, punitive behavioural interventions and the management of the behaviour based on avoidance rather than therapeutic risk taking. In turn, this can lead to abusive practice.

Care and treatment in cases where a person displays challenging behaviour within secure forensic settings should follow the guiding principles outlined in Chapter 1 of the Mental Health Act Code of Practice (DH, 2008).

Communication-based interventions should be promoted over reactive and restrictive ones. Care and treatment should be focused on improving and developing pro-social skills that will reduce the need for challenging behaviour, rather than solely on the management of the behaviour when it happens.

Care and treatment should also seek to reduce the underlying causational factors, as without the reduction in these factors there will be little reduction in the level of challenging behaviour. Inability to do this will lead to a negative cycle of behaviour and management, behaviour and management, which may make the challenging behaviour worse over time.

Implementing person-centred care and promoting participation

Managing boundaries

Managing therapeutic boundaries in difficult interactions

In order to promote individuals' recovery and to provide a safe and emotionally secure environment, it is very important that we manage therapeutic boundaries. However, managing boundaries in a secure forensic mental health setting can present many issues.

Think about any incidents of challenging behaviour you have witnessed at work. How does your service manage challenging behaviours – are they the best approach?

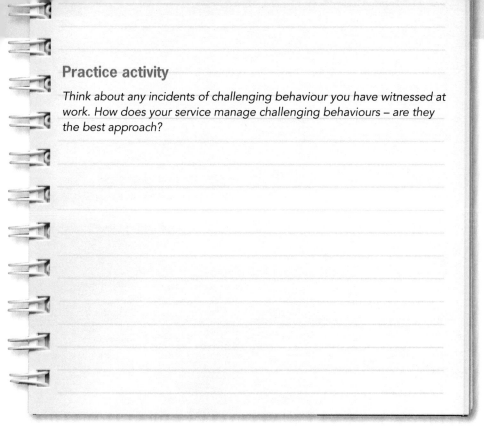

Imagine you are having a conversation with an individual in the day area: a colleague interjects with their 'thoughts' – only to help, of course. Or, talking to someone who is upset, another individual shouts, 'Don't be a silly bitch and grow up.'

We do not manage therapeutic boundaries in isolation. It is far more complex to manage them in a secure forensic environment simply because it is a 'public space'. (Access is limited to the patient and staffing groups admitted, but it is still a very public environment.)

There are a number of simple things that can make management a lot easier.

- Cast your mind back to school: you are in the classroom and a teacher belittles you for getting an answer wrong in front of your classmates, how did this make you feel? Do not attempt an intervention with an individual in front of their peers that could be perceived as belittling. They have to live with their peers and manage the ward dynamics.

- Choose a suitable place to have a conversation with the individual, if there is need for another staff member to be present, brief them as to what their role is.

- If a colleague is in conversation with an individual about an issue, do not interrupt with your thoughts. If your colleague is not at risk then don't intervene, your intervention may escalate risk.

- If an individual is excited, overly agitated, irritable or angry, do not expect them to:
    - listen to a long rational list of what you want them to do
    - be 'responsible for their actions'
    - follow their care plan.

Imagine how you would feel if you felt angry and someone asked you to, 'calm down, dear'. It could antagonise the situation.

Give the person:

- space to get things off their chest
- respect
- time to calm down

- access to a quieter space
- access to an activity that will divert them.

Interventions are not about power, control or being 'one-up', but about the therapeutic use of self.

Once the person is in a calmer and more receptive frame of mind, then you can talk to them about the situation. For example, you could say: 'Do you remember yesterday when you called me a stupid bitch? How do you think that made me feel?'

Managing boundaries is also about managing your environment. You should:

- keep noise down to an appropriate level
- ensure offenders have access to fresh air and exercise

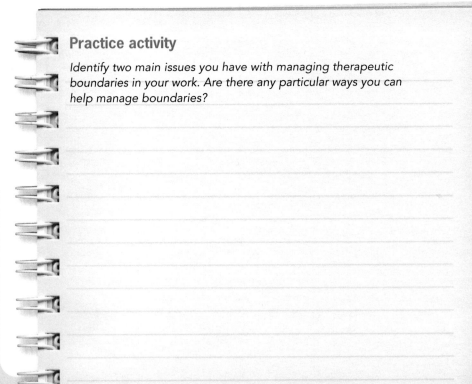

Practice activity

Identify two main issues you have with managing therapeutic boundaries in your work. Are there any particular ways you can help manage boundaries?

- keep your environment safe, clean and tidy
- ensure individuals have access to activities
- ensure that there is a meaningful structure to the day
- reduce the number of 'rules' – arguing over rules can take the focus away from therapeutic activity.

Thinking activity

Think about a situation in which you found it difficult to manage your communication/behaviour when working with an offender with a mental disorder. What did you say or do?

Managing self in difficult interactions

Individuals within secure forensic settings will present with complex, difficult and often challenging behaviour. They may antagonise you or 'press your buttons' in order to test out your reaction.

Many of the people we support have experienced negative reactions in their lives. Some think they deserve it and some have come to expect it. Pushing our buttons is not always a way to manipulate or hurt us, it can just be a way for people to gauge whether we can work with them, keeping them safe and emotionally secure. They are testing us to see whether we are as fair, trustworthy, honest, reliable and firm as we say we are.

How we manage ourselves and our communication is very important; the people we support have a lot of time to observe our behaviour and, just like everybody else, they will make judgments.

In managing ourselves we must be aware of our impact on the patient group, the response and reaction to the way that we communicate.

We must be aware of our:

- body language – our facial expressions, posture and gestures make up the largest portion of our communication
- intonation – the tone/pitch of our voice
- content – the actual message, the words we use.

Before any verbal intervention, give yourself time to take in the person's tone of voice and body language, whilst being aware of your surroundings and how you are feeling. Self-awareness is the key in the management of self. Think before you speak!

Managing our communication

It is imperative that you are aware of your communication and its impact. Remember to engage your brain before you open your mouth!

Conflict resolution

Communication in conflict resolution

Conflict resolution is about managing potential and existing friction between two or more people. Friction causes heat that can ignite into a fire. Our job is to eradicate or to reduce friction, to stop the situation getting hotter and reduce the likelihood of a conflict getting out of hand.

It is vital that you know the individuals you support and your colleagues. An awareness of the environment and self-awareness are also key. Self-awareness means understanding the impact of your language (content, intonation and non-verbal) on the other people involved.

Using an adapted version of Eric Berne's transactional analysis model (Figure 2.1), we can briefly look at how we engage in conflict resolution.

Berne said that everyone has three alter ego states:

1. Parent
2. Adult
3. Child

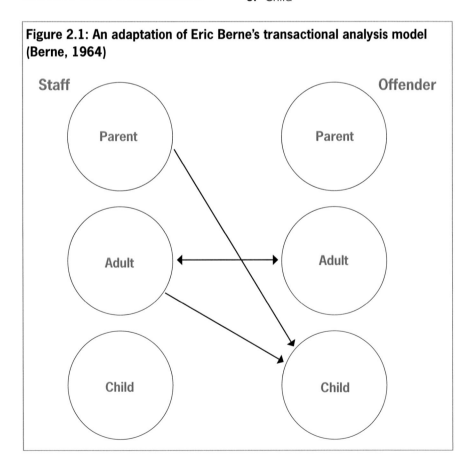

Figure 2.1: An adaptation of Eric Berne's transactional analysis model (Berne, 1964)

Berne suggested that when we communicate we do so in one of these three states.

The best relationship for interactions between two adults is obviously adult-to-adult and this is the one that should be encouraged at all times.

Often a person's behaviour can regress (not necessarily in a childish way), and they become aggressive and challenging. Their behaviour will have regressed to the 'child' mode, as illustrated in Figure 2.1. (Do not interpret this to mean that the person is childish, childlike or like a 'big kid'.)

It does not help to move into the role of the parent, as this tends to take one of two major forms: critical or nurturing, neither of which is of use in conflict resolution.

Critical communication may push the person into feeling 'spoken down to', treated like a child and even angrier. Nurturing communication may make the person feel smothered, patronised and even angrier.

You must also take care not to slip into child mode through verbal ping-pong: 'I told you,' 'No you didn't,' 'Yes I did' etc.

Remain the adult and allow the person space to work through things. You can be in control without being controlling.

In resolving or reducing conflict in your work with offenders, it important that you manage boundaries, manage yourself and your own responses, use effective communication and avoid

Thinking activity

How do you know when people are engaged in conflict? What is their body language, facial expression, tone of voice and what language do they use?

turning interventions with offenders into a 'battle of wills'.

Reflective practice

Reflective practice is important in ensuring that care and treatment is person-centred and that patient participation is promoted.

The reflective cycle

There are four steps to follow when using the reflective cycle to solve problems.

Step one: identify the issue

It is the responsibility of the person in supervision to bring a subject to reflect on. If the issue is vague, then it will need to be clarified. The person facilitating the reflective practice must, through questioning, clarify the issue using questions such as:

- what?
- when?
- how?
- who?

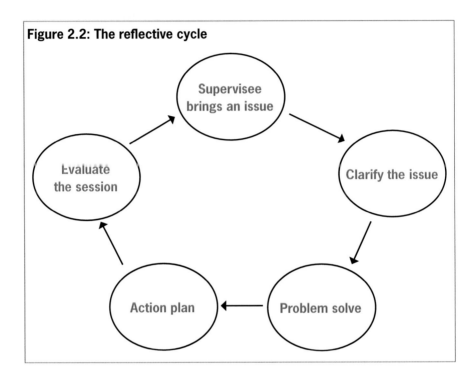

Figure 2.2: The reflective cycle

- Supervisee brings an issue
- Clarify the issue
- Problem solve
- Action plan
- Evaluate the session

(Avoid 'why' questions. For example, 'Why did you become upset?' does not aid the identification of the issue as it is not focused enough.)

This stage of the process can almost act as a mini reflective cycle and clarifying the issue might help bring resolution.

Step two: start problem solving

Once the issue is clarified, begin to problem solve.

Again use questioning. For example:

- Is your approach helping or not?
- Is it part of the person's condition?
- What happens next?
- What does the person like doing?

- Does the person respond differently to other members of staff?
- How does it make you feel?
- Can you think of other ways of doing it?

Through questioning, the facilitator will recognise what is at the root of the issue for the staff member and what is necessary to move the reflective practice on.

- If it is a lack of knowledge, then bring the information into the process.
- If it is a lack of understanding, then guide the supervisee.
- If it is a lack of experience, support the supervisee and ensure that they

feel safe and that they are safe to practise.

- If it is a poor attitude, challenge the supervisee to explore how that may impact on individuals in their care.

Step three: action planning

Talk through how the supervisee is going to put what has been discussed into action and how they are going to evaluate this action.

Step four: evaluation

Talk through how the reflection went.

- Did it help?
- What went well?

- What didn't go well?
- How could it be improved?

Arrange the next reflective practice.

Write up reflective practice notes.

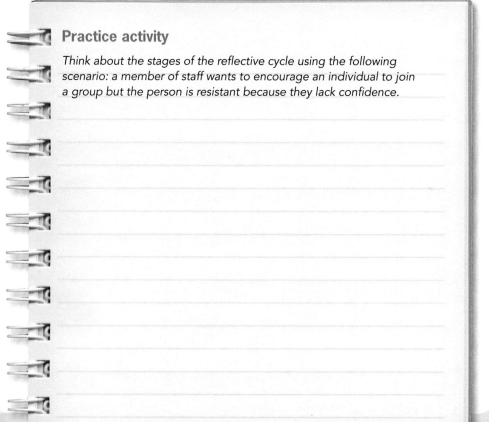

Practice activity

Think about the stages of the reflective cycle using the following scenario: a member of staff wants to encourage an individual to join a group but the person is resistant because they lack confidence.

Thinking activity

How often do you make use of reflective practice in your role?

- medication management
- daily living skills
- communication skills
- how to manage their drug/alcohol issues.

(The list above is not exhaustive.)

We need to understand our role in this education process and think about how we can act as role models. We role model behaviour and should of course demonstrate pro-social behaviour that benefits others. This means we have to manage ourselves and manage our therapeutic boundaries.

The recovery model

The recovery approach

A holistic (whole person) approach is the foundation of any recovery model, and it is an approach that aims to enable social inclusion. Any individual within a secure environment is excluded from society by being detained. They are also excluded by the nature of their disorder.

A recovery model will seek to increase an offender's ability to manage their behaviour in order to increase self-empowerment and autonomy, improve the quality of their life and to help them achieve their personal goals and ambitions.

A large part of any recovery model is that of education – not education through individuals sitting in a classroom but, for example, through learning about:

- life and social skills
- how to manage their problems
- their illness/diagnosis
- how to manage their anger

Recovery tools

There are specific recovery tools that can support the recovery process.

The recovery star

The recovery star has domains covering aspects of a person's life, including living skills, work and self-esteem. Individuals should set their own goals in each area and be supported in achieving them. Therapeutic risk taking should be an enabling factor. They can then use the recovery star to measure their own progress through recovery with the help of healthcare professionals, family members and carers.

Recovery should offer hope and the recovery star will enable individuals to measure and to build on their progress.

For more information see: http://www.mhpf.org.uk/programmes/mental-health-and-recovery/the-recoverystar

WRAP
(Wellness Recovery Action Planning)

WRAP is an American recovery tool that supports individuals in developing their own wellness recovery action plan by setting realistic goals and identifying what help they need to achieve them. WRAP helps to highlight what makes and keeps individuals well and what puts their mental health at risk. It also looks at what support and help theywill need if they become unwell.

For more information see: http://www.mentalhealthrecovery.com/

DREEM
(Developing Recovery Enhancing Environments Measure)

This is very much a research and outcome measure. Its purpose is to assess how 'recovery oriented' the environment is. It is a self-reported, user-friendly tool, which works by asking people questions about their recovery and the process supporting it.

For more information see: http://www.recoverydevon.co.uk/download/DREEM%20total%20dft4%20no%20tc.pdf

It is very important to remember that many offenders are not at the engagement stage when they are first admitted to secure forensic settings and may resist care and treatment or refuse to engage with any programme. This does not exclude them from the need for involvement in their care, positive role modelling or a recovery-based environment.

Maintaining person-centred records

Recording safe and supportive observation and engagement

Observation of individuals within secure forensic mental health environments is a difficult task at the best of times. The occasions when observation is most needed are normally the times when individuals find being observed the most difficult and challenging. Observation must then be undertaken with safe and supportive engagement in mind.

Effective observation

Observation at its worst can be nothing more than a mechanistic conveyor belt of checks and rechecks. It can be a task that is seen more as a punishment – for both staff and offenders with mental disorders – than as a therapeutic intervention aimed at ensuring the safety of the individual and others.

Observation is an activity which is based on knowing:

- risk factors
- offenders with mental disorders
- the environment
- ward dynamics
- where you are – are you in line of sight; do your colleagues know where you are?
- where your colleagues are – have they left the unit without telling anybody?
- policy and procedures
- trigger factors eg:
  - a telephone call from a relative
  - admission of a new offender with a mental disorder
- behavioural indicators eg:
  - deterioration in personal hygiene
  - social withdrawal
- not taking medication (this is both a trigger factor and a behavioural indicator).

Observation and the ability to engage in a safe and supportive manner cannot be effective without the relevant information and an understanding of the factors outlined above. Imagine if you walked onto the unit for the first time and somebody asked you to watch the patients. You might be able to look at the patients, but you would not know exactly what you were being asked to look for or how to engage safely. You and the individuals in the unit would be at risk.

You will need to engage with all of your senses, not just by looking. In order to observe effectively you also need to engage with the patients – just sitting watching is not very good practice. Individuals may find being observed difficult and feeling that people are just 'watching over them' can exacerbate the situation.

Remember that respect and dignity also play a big part in safe and supportive engagement. For example, at times we may have to observe/engage whilst people take care of their personal hygiene needs. These can be embarrassing situations, and special care needs to be taken at these times. Often we will also have to observe private activities, such as family visits, and this will need to be handled sensitively.

Each of the people in our care is an individual and will respond differently to different people. You need to be aware of your own relationship with the person and how it affects your engagement with them.

Levels of engagement

Level 1

All of the patients are on general observation (level 1) all of the time. This involves determining and understanding:

- where they are
- what they are doing
- who they are with
- what risk items they have access to
- how they are responding to their environment
- whether there are any changes in the dynamics on the ward.

Individuals who are not presenting risk or who are managed safely within the unit will be under general observation, with recording of their behaviour/activity completed every hour.

Sometimes an individual's observations may need to be enhanced; this is normally when they are presenting a greater level of risk to themselves or others, or if they are vulnerable to risk.

Level 2

Level 2 observation requires an increase in the recording of an individual's behaviour and activity to every 10 or 15 minutes, or done randomly during the hour. It does not mean that you can forget the person between 'five minute checks' – it only takes 10–12 seconds to die from self-ligation so this could prove fatal. Common sense and knowing the people you support are key.

Level 3

Level 3 observation is 'within line of sight'. The individual does not require 'close' observation but due to the nature of the risk needs constant and discrete observation.

Level 4

Level 4 observation is 'within arm's length'. It is the most invasive level of observation and can be seen as the worst 'job' to do. Staff engagement on this level of observation needs to be highly attuned and it can be very tiring. For this reason and according to policy, a member of staff should only carry out this level of observation for a maximum of two hours.

Level 4 observation is not about confining an individual to a chair and excluding them; it is about managing the observation whilst engaging the individual. Sometimes, due to the nature and degree of risk, the person's access to certain objects and areas may be restricted. As stated, this is not about excluding them from activities, but managing what they can have access to safely, as far as possible with the participation of the individual.

Thinking activity

Think about a busy mealtime in your service; how easy is it to observe everything that happens while still engaging with individuals and ensuring that everyone is safe?

Safe and supportive engagement

In order to be able to safely engage with a patient group and offer active support, we need to know certain information about them and their environment.

Patient information eg:

- What are the behavioural indicators?
  - What are the trigger factors?
  - What works?
  - What doesn't work?
- What are the risk factors?

Environmental information eg:

- Where are the patients?

Effective engagement in observation is all about mitigating the potential negative effects, reducing the level of intrusion and maintaining the individual's privacy, dignity and respect.

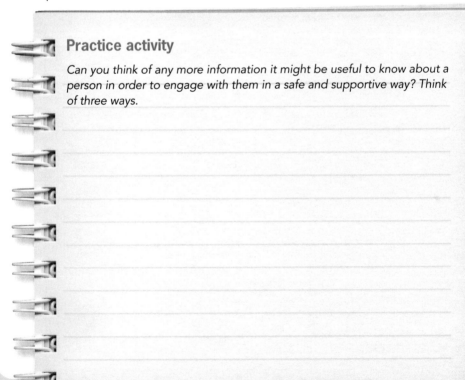

Practice activity

Can you think of any more information it might be useful to know about a person in order to engage with them in a safe and supportive way? Think of three ways.

- Where are your colleagues?
- Where are you?
- What are the ward dynamics?

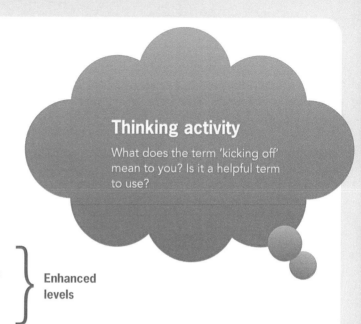

Thinking activity

What does the term 'kicking off' mean to you? Is it a helpful term to use?

1. General observation
2. Random observation
3. Line of sight
4. Arm's length

} Enhanced levels

Recording safe and supportive engagement

Avoiding jargon and negative language

Most cultures have their own language, their own way of expressing things; secure forensic mental health environments are the same. The problem is that the language we use can creep into our record keeping and it can also affect how individuals are perceived.

Negative and jargonised language can adversely affect risk assessment. For example, what does the word 'settled' mean in somebody's clinical records? Settled is an unhelpful word which is often used as shorthand for non-presentation of negative behaviour. This can mean that there is no clinical record of positive behaviour. Settled is also a non-descriptor and holds no clinical validity; therefore it does not support effective clinical and risk assessment.

Your records are a way for you to evidence your practice as well as describing the care/treatment of the person and their:

- mood
- mental state
- engagement
- activity
- social skills
- life skills
- risk factors etc.

The recording we do today becomes part of the person's history. The notes we write should objectively demonstrate:

- what we see
- what we did
- what the individual did
- the context of the situation eg:
  - who was involved
  - the dynamics at the time
  - the time of day
  - trigger factors
  - the causational factors
  - the outcome – how it was resolved
- what we 'hear' eg:
  - the words used
  - the tone of voice used
  - body language.

Use clear descriptors to share the situation with the audience you are telling the story to. (Section 4 covers the people who may read clinical case notes.)

We must take care not to use inappropriate custodial language, for example, 'sharps' for cutlery, 'contraband' for restricted items, 'sharps time' for meals, 'fresh air' for time outside etc. Describing individuals according to their 'behaviour' – for example, 'she's the self-harmer' – is not good practice as it causes you to lose sight of the person. This is not the language of recovery, but the language of being 'locked up', the language of exclusion.

We need to use the language of inclusion and participation, for example:

- 'in conversation with…'
- 'whilst we were … we…'
- 'my intervention was aimed at…'
- 'I offered … and she stated that…'
- 'his manner was … and his tone of voice suggested that…'
- 'it was the first time that … managed to achieve…'.

The majority of the entries in an individual's clinical records are about negative situations or occasions when the person has done something 'wrong'.

This needs to be balanced with the times when they have managed situations well and acted appropriately. Remember, clinical records are a window into our practice.

Regulatory and policy documentation

The service you work within will be subject to various local, practice-based record keeping policies. It is imperative that you are familiar and up-to-date with these policies and their requirements. You must also make sure that any recorded information meets with the CQC's requirements.

Care Quality Commission (CQC) standards

Any provider of health and social care, whether public, private or voluntary (charitable or non-profit making), must

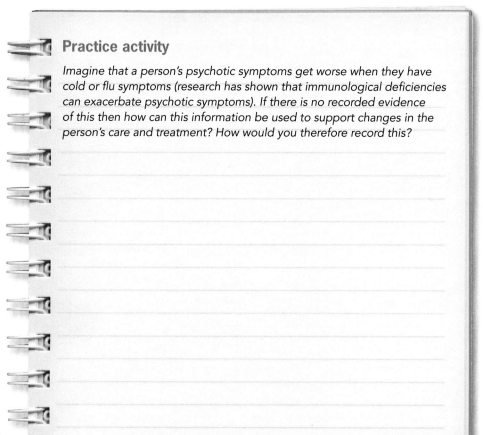

Practice activity

Imagine that a person's psychotic symptoms get worse when they have cold or flu symptoms (research has shown that immunological deficiencies can exacerbate psychotic symptoms). If there is no recorded evidence of this then how can this information be used to support changes in the person's care and treatment? How would you therefore record this?

Regulation 13: Management of medicines

Regulation 15: Safety and suitability of premises

Regulation 16: Safety, availability and suitability of equipment

Suitability of staffing

Regulation 21: Requirements relating to workers

Regulation 22: Staffing

Regulation 23: Supporting workers

meet 16 key standards. This means that all employees must ensure that their practice supports the standards outlined below.

Involvement and information

Regulation 17: Respecting and involving service users

Regulation 18: Consent to care and treatment

Personalised care, treatment and support

Regulation 9: Care and welfare of service users

Regulation 14: Meeting nutritional needs

Regulation 24: Co-operating with other providers

Safeguarding and safety

Regulation 11: Safeguarding service users from abuse

Regulation 12: Cleanliness and infection control

Quality and management

Regulation 10: Assessing and monitoring the quality of service provision

Regulation 19: Complaints

Regulation 20: Records

The CQC has the power to inspect any service provider and can, if the standards are not met, ask the service to improve or, in case of serious breach of the standards, close the service down.

Practice activity

Download and read the Nursing and Midwifery Council Record Keeping Guidelines (available from: http://www.nmc-uk.org/Documents/NMC-Publications/NMC-Record-Keeping-Guidance.pdf). How can you record information accurately and in line with the policy?

Assessing risk and recording information

Introduction

This section covers the role of risk assessment and management in a secure forensic mental health setting, with particular reference to your role. It covers relational security and how to perform observation while maintaining safe and supportive engagement. It will help you to understand the principles of positive engagement and the communication skills needed for risk assessment, risk management and recovery.

The provision of ongoing risk assessment for individuals detained in secure forensic mental health settings is an essential function. It must be undertaken in an effective and efficient manner with a well-informed and trained workforce. Risk assessment should be meaningful, evidence-based and inter-professional. It should be carried out with the participation of the person and significant others, including family, friends and carers, and use clinical and actuarial assessments while also ensuring that it is holistic. This section outlines the nature and practice of risk assessment and encourages learners to identify strategies for effectively managing risk.

The nature and practice of risk assessment in secure forensic mental health settings

Risk defined

Risk is when a situation presents the possibility of something dangerous or harmful happening. For example, walking along the top of a high cliff is a potentially dangerous situation. There is a risk of you falling.

Assessing risk

There are factors that will increase your risk of falling over the edge of the cliff, for example:

- proximity – the nearer you get, the more the risk increases (being closer to the edge of the cliff may also influence the other factors)
- your state of mind
- weather conditions (eg. fog, high winds)
- alcohol consumption
- drug use
- erosion.

There are also factors that will reduce your risk of falling over the edge of the cliff. These could include risk reduction and prevention measures, for example:

- fencing preventing access
- signs pointing out the danger
- education to teach people about the dangers of being near a cliff edge.

In order to ensure that the reduction and prevention measures are going to be effective, an assessment of the risk needs to be undertaken.

There are several stages to any risk assessment:

1. Identification and recognition of the 'danger'
2. Gathering of the relevant information
3. Analysis of the information
4. Redefining the 'danger' if the analysis has highlighted other factors to consider
5. Identification of the specific risk

Risk management

After assessing the risk, the next step is the risk management process. Risk management involves developing plans to manage any potentially dangerous or harmful situations and deciding who will be responsible for implementing the actions.

Implementation

Risk management often fails at the point of implementation. Thinking again about the cliff example: if the decision had been made to put up signs on the seaward side of the coastal path but the person implementing the plan decided to put them on the landward side ('so as not to spoil the view'), then the management of the risk would be compromised, with an increased chance of someone falling over the edge of the cliff.

Risk assessment and risk management

Risk management can also fail because of poor risk assessment. Risk assessment must be based

on reliable, objective and clearly documented information. You are involved in collecting this information, and therefore in risk assessment, from the moment that you enter the secure forensic mental health setting.

Risk assessment requires you to observe and reflect upon:

- your environment
- your patient group
- where you are
- where your colleagues are
- factors that might change any of the above.

The environment

This is about the physical aspects of the place where you are working, for example, locks, doors, windows, broken chairs, etc., as well as the ambience, for example, noise levels, lighting and the 'mood' on the ward/unit.

The patient group

Understanding your patient group requires you to observe and reflect on:

- appearance and behaviour
- mood and affect
- speech

- thought
- perception
- cognition
- insight.

Where you are

It is very important that you know where you are and that you have not placed yourself in a position of risk or vulnerability. Ideally you should ensure that you are in line of sight of your colleagues, and, if not, that they know where you are, who you are with and how long you will be. Do not become isolated! The risks of becoming isolated could include, assault, accusations, being taken hostage, and complaints. If you are 'alone' with an individual, ensure that the situation has been risk assessed and documented.

For the same reasons, you should work as a team, ensuring safety. Do not leave the area without informing your colleagues where you are going.

Your role in risk assessment

Your role is to observe, reflect upon and share information verbally and in written form. The information that they share becomes an active part of risk assessment both in the present and in the future management, treatment and care of the person.

You cannot risk assess effectively:

- if you do not interact with the people you are supporting

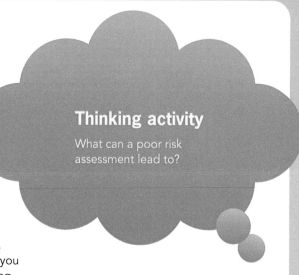

Thinking activity

What can a poor risk assessment lead to?

- if you do not know the people you are supporting eg:
  - trigger factors
  - behavioural indicators
- if you do not know your physical environment
- if you are not aware of how you are feeling and the potential impact of your behaviour
- if you have not had a proper hand-over or if you have not been informed of possible risk issues
- if you do not know the inherent risks on the ward eg:
  - cutlery
  - CDs
  - blind-spots
  - ligature points
  - pens.

Environmental factors in risk assessment

In a secure forensic mental health setting you should know what the risk factors are. If you do not know, you should find out. This may mean conducting room searches: 'Where has that pen gone?', 'Has that individual secreted any tablets?' It may also mean searches of the wider environment or patient searches.

Your role in these activities is to ensure that they are completed properly, in line with policy, and with due respect for the person's privacy, dignity and personal belongings.

Practice activity

Look around the room you are in and identify any risk factors. Think about floors, tripping hazards, blocked walkways, unmarked fire exits, blind spots.

Environmental risk factors

The physical environment eg:

- doors
- locks/keys
- pens/cutlery
- blind spots.

Ambience eg:

- noise level
- light
- air quality.

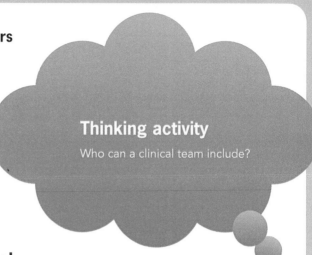

Thinking activity

Who can a clinical team include?

The role of the clinical team in risk assessment

The role of the clinical team – normally under a responsible clinician, for example, a psychiatrist/psychologist/nurse etc. – is to ensure that an individual's care, treatment and management is 'appropriate' to their need and to the least level of restriction (DH, 2008).

The team has a further responsibility to ensure that this care, treatment and management is in line with the legal, ethical and best practice requirements.

This includes keeping the person safe and protecting others from harm. In order to ensure that this happens they need 'good' information on which to base their assessment of risk.

Risk may be in relation to:

- harm to self
- harm to others
- self-neglect
- a decline in mental state
- physical aspects of care
- social aspects of care

- offence-related issues
- drug and alcohol abuse
- social factors
- challenging behaviour
- environmental changes
- ward dynamics
- effectiveness of care.

(This list is not exhaustive.)

The clinical team will then formulate the person's care, treatment and management plans. Poor information will lead to poor care, treatment and management outcomes.

The clinical team may use other forms of risk and clinical assessments to gather information. Tools may include:

- Short-Term Assessment of Risk and Treatability (START) (Webster *et al*, 2004)
- Beck Depression Inventory (BDI-II) (Beck *et al*, 1996)

Key learning point

Risk management must be based on informed and informative risk assessment.

- KGV symptom severity scale (Krawiecka *et al*, 1977)
- Historical, Clinical, Risk Management-20 (HCR-20) violence prediction tool (Webster *et al*, 1997).

Who can be in a clinical team?

The clinical team can include:

- occupational therapists
- social workers
- psychiatrists
- nurses
- psychologists
- speech and language therapists.

Risk management within a secure forensic mental health environment

Risk management is based on effective risk assessment and information sharing.

Risk management covers the management of:

- the environment
- your own feelings and emotions
- interventions and interactions with the patient group
- the individual's and the patient group's challenging behaviour

- the individual's mental disorder and effects of symptomatology on themselves and others
- interactions and interventions of the team
- the individual's interactions with other offenders, staff members, family, friends and other professionals.

This should be reflected in clear and realistic care and management plans which guide the staff team in how to manage risk behaviours. They should outline:

- what works
- what doesn't work
- how to approach the person
- diversions
- the person's wishes as to how they want to be managed in crisis
- the steps to be taken to reduce risk, not just the steps to 'manage' it
- any restrictions (to the least restriction principle)
- any environmental factors
- any social factors
- any historical factors that may impact on the management of risk
- fair boundary setting.

Risk management also requires the provision of a fair and open structure to the day. The structure should be, as far as is possible, negotiated through user involvement forums, such as ward meetings. It should not be confused with control – a controlling environment can be imposed, punitive and overly restrictive. It is possible to be 'in control' without being controlling.

Risk management can be either risk-averse or risk-taking. A risk-averse management structure could appear 'controlling' as it may impinge on people's rights and restrict what activities individuals can participate in. It may also seem like a safe strategy, which can paradoxically increase the level of risk.

The purpose of risk management is to enable recovery while keeping the person and others safe. Therefore, risk management must not be based on total risk avoidance, but on properly assessed, therapeutic risk taking. If you are risk averse, the individual cannot be therapeutically challenged.

It is everybody's role to be involved and informed, and to share information related to the management of risk.

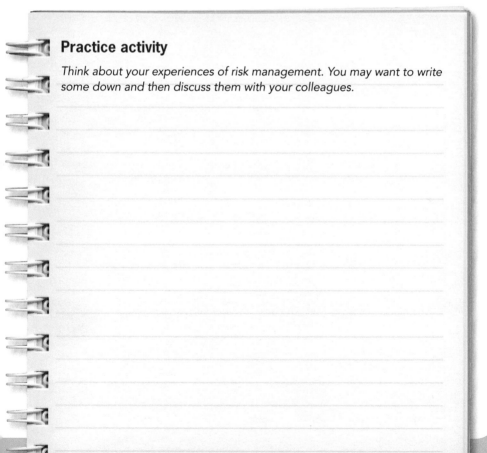

Practice activity

Think about your experiences of risk management. You may want to write some down and then discuss them with your colleagues.

It is also essential for the individual to be involved in the assessment and management of their risk behaviours. It aids engagement in their care and treatment and motivation to progress along the road to recovery.

While controlling risk can involve preventing people from doing things so that any potential risk is removed, effective risk management supports people to participate in activities safely by minimising risk.

Relational security

Relational security plays a key role in risk management as it is through knowing the individuals in our care that we can build a therapeutic relationship with them. (Note: A therapeutic relationship should not be mistaken for one of friendship, and should not be considered in the context of 'us and them'.)

Relational security should demonstrate that to some degree you are aware of and can understand how the individual feels 'inside'. For example, you might want to know the answers to some of the following questions.

- What is going on for them?
- Is there an anniversary coming up?
- Are they suffering from flashbacks?
- Are they being haunted by bad memories?
- Are they being influenced negatively by their peers?
- Are they being bullied?
- Are they finding change difficult?
- Are they suffering from side-effects of medication?
- What is the impact of their mental disorder?

Relational security means that we will notice changes in a person's behaviour and respond therapeutically to them. If we cannot help then we need to ensure that someone who can is aware that action is needed. We will share information with the clinical team and change things if they need to be changed. Observation and understanding alone are not enough; if we do not do something to help we are failing in our duty of care.

Relational security is about being active in observation, communication, and the care and treatment of the patient group.

You can download a PDF about relational security from:

www.rcpsych.ac.uk/pdf/ Relational%20Security%20BH.pdf

Thinking activity

What skills do you think you need to implement relational security?

Observation in safe and supportive engagement

Observation in safe and supportive engagement is an essential part of risk management. Sharing information is important in the management of risk. It prevents knowledge gaps, ensures clear and unambiguous handovers, ensures that the relevant members of staff have the information they need to keep themselves and others safe and enables effective risk assessment and management to take place.

Mitigating risk

Risk assessment and management are about reducing/preventing harm. There are things that we do that can:

- reduce the risk of harm
- increase the risk of harm.

We need to do those things that reduce the risk!

Thinking activity

Think about the information you need to know in order to provide effective observation. What do you need to share with others following an observation?

Some examples of risk reducing factors include:

- encouraging the individual's participation in their care and treatment
- listening to and acting upon the individual's advance wishes and statements
- a safe and supportive environment
- clear, open and honest communication
- provision of meaningful activities
  - good risk assessment practice – well documented and effectively shared information relating to risk assessment.

Some examples of factors that enhance risk include:

- punitive restrictions
- boredom
- poor communication
- an unsafe environment

Thinking activity

Think about some factors that can enhance risk and some factors that can reduce risk.

Practice activity

Read through the following scenario and identify factors that could increase the level of risk. Then think about some strategies that could reduce the level of risk.

It is a very busy day on a 12-bed unit catering for 11 female detainees with the predominant diagnosis of personality disorder.

A new admission is expected in about three hours' time.

An individual has self-harmed and is very distressed. She does not need hospital attention.

You have a fairly new member of staff working who is a registered nurse and does not yet know all of the detainees, policies and procedures, or where everything is.

The registered nurse is the only one on the ward, as there is a Care Programme Approach (CPA) meeting going on and the charge nurse/ team leader is attending.

It is pouring down with rain.

You are with five other members of your team; thankfully you and everyone apart from the new member of staff are experienced and know the detainees and the ward routine.

- a patronising care regime
- poor documentation or failure to share information relating to risk.

Encourage and support the participation of individuals in risk assessment and management

Thinking activity

What are some of the ways you can encourage engagement? What will hinder engagement?

Engagement

Patients within secure forensic mental health services are detained; they are not there on a voluntary basis. This very simple statement highlights that for many of the people we support, the idea of their own engagement may be very alien. Why should they engage with us when they have been 'forced' to be there? However, effective risk assessment and management requires the engagement of the offender with a mental disorder – their recovery depends on it.

In order to encourage an individual's engagement in the risk assessment and management process, it can help to:

- build a therapeutic relationship
- demonstrate honest and trustworthy communication and behaviour
- provide relevant information
- ask the person their views and wishes, and when possible acting on them.

Do not let an individual's attendance at an activity be mistaken for engagement in a therapeutic activity. Attendance only requires that the person is present, but engagement is a genuine and meaningful interaction with a therapeutic outcome. Risk issues, especially around offence behaviour, can be missed simply because an individual is attending an activity and displaying socially acceptable behaviour.

Communication in risk assessment and management

In order to enable individuals to engage effectively in risk assessment and management, we need to ensure that our communication, either in verbal or written form, is clear, unambiguous, honest, and that it provides a basis for safe and supportive engagement.

If the staff–patient relationship does not have a foundation of trust, then risk assessment and management may be seen to be 'done to' the person rather than 'with' them.

The communication required in order for us to accurately assess risk may be seen as 'intrusive', as it may require us to ask questions about the person's past and the reasons for some of the things they have done. This could increase the level of risk if handled at the wrong time or in the wrong way. It is sometimes better to step away from a conversation if you do not have the skills, knowledge and ability to deal with these questions sensitively.

Many of the individuals we support do not have the language to express how they feel and find that talking about it increases their anxiety. Anxiety can increase the chance of risk behaviour occurring. Because of this, staff members may not talk about issues because they are fearful of provoking a negative reaction. This can lead to challenging behaviour 'recycling', rather than being managed safely.

Communication around these issues does need to happen, but in ways that minimise the individual's anxiety.

Approaches to communication

There are many different ways you can approach communication with the individuals you support. This could even mean using things like:

- poetry
- art
- storytelling
- examples from soap operas or gossip magazines
- DVD or video.

It is important to create the right 'space' for people to feel safe to talk.

Think about:

- the room
- the noise level
- who else is around
- the questions you will ask and how you will ask them
- the information you need
- what indicators there might be that you need to give the person some space
- what to do with information that it is not within your experience to deal with
- pre-planning support should the person become distressed.

Try new ways of engaging with the people you support, based on your relationship with them and ongoing assessment of risk. Share with them that you want to try something new and ask for their feedback on how they think it went.

The skills necessary to share risk information with colleagues, family members, carers and the individual detained within the legal framework

People who may potentially read clinical records include:

- social workers
- visiting professionals
- the offender with a mental disorder
- psychologists
- psychiatrists
- occupational therapists

- unpatronising
- honest
- enabling.

Sharing verbal information in regards to clinical and risk issues is always more effective when supported by written evidence that includes clear observations, contextual information and recommendations for an individual's future care, treatment and management.

The language that you use when talking about risk is very important, and in order to be accurate in your recording you need to have a basic knowledge of the subjects that apply to the patient group within your care – a knowledge of the subject of self-harm for example, combined with knowledge of the person, will enable you to more accurately describe risks relating to this.

- nurses
- clinical specialists eg. drug or alcohol workers
- advocates.

Verbal communication skills in risk assessment and management

In order to share information relating to risk with someone else, it is very important to know the audience that you are going to share it with. This does not mean 'dumbing down' information; it means ensuring that information is communicated in the most appropriate and effective way to get the message across.

Verbal communication relating to risk should be:

- knowledge-based
- person-centred
- accurate
- both informed and informing
- communicated in a way that meets the needs of the audience – whilst the information remains the same, the sharer of the information must provide it in such a way that the receiver can understand it:

Written and communication skills in risk assessment and management

Clear and effective written records not only help to protect the welfare of the patient group, they also protect the healthcare professional's practice. Remember, what is written today becomes part of the person's history and part of future risk assessments. Good record keeping promotes:

- high standards of clinical care
- continuity of care
- better communication and dissemination of information between members of the clinical team
- an accurate account of the treatment, and care planning and delivery

- the ability to detect problems, such as changes in the person's condition, at an early stage
- the concept of confidentiality.

Records include:
- medication charts
- daily clinical records
- care plans
- management plans
- observation records
- reports
- physical care records/charts
- assessments
- letters to other professionals.

This covers both handwritten and electronic records.

(The above list is by no means exhaustive.)

Content and style

There are a number of factors that contribute to effective record keeping. Patient records should:

- be factual, consistent and accurate
- be written as soon as possible after an event has occurred, providing current information on the care and condition of the person
- be written clearly and in such a manner that the text cannot be erased or deleted without a record of the change
- be written in such a manner that any justifiable alterations or additions are identifiable and made in such a way that the original entry can still be read
- be accurately dated, timed and signed, with the signature printed alongside the first entry where there is a written record, or, for electronic records,
- clearly attributed to a named person in an identifiable role
- not include jargon, meaningless phrases, irrelevant speculation or offensive subjective statements
- be readable on photocopies
- be written, wherever possible, with the participation of the person
- be written in terms that the individual can understand
- be consecutive
- not be left until the end of the shift
- identify any problems that have arisen and the action that was taken to rectify them
- provide clear evidence of the intervention planned, the decisions made, the care delivered and the information shared.

Thinking activity

How could the way you write clinical records affect an individual's future?

All clinical documentation should reflect the Mental Health Act (2007) (MHA) guiding principles.

Sharing information

Information may need to be shared in different ways depending on the audience. Information, by its definition, needs to inform; anything that is vague, ill-defined or not evidence-based ceases to be informative.

Thinking activity

How can you effectively share information?

Legal compliance

Patient records are sometimes called into evidence in order to investigate a complaint at a local level, for criminal proceedings or for Coroners' Court. Healthcare professionals have both a professional and a legal duty of care, and legal accountability under the MHA and the MCA. Record keeping should therefore be able to demonstrate:

- a full account of risk assessment and the care that has been planned and provided
- relevant information about the condition of the person at any given time
- the measures taken by the member of staff to respond to the individual's needs
- evidence that the member of staff has understood and honoured their duty of care, that all reasonable steps have been taken to care for the person, and that any actions or omissions on the part of the member of staff have not compromised the individual's safety in any way

- a record of any arrangements that have been made for the continuing care of an individual.

The frequency of entries will be determined by clinical judgment and local standards. Members of staff should make more frequent entries for individuals who:

- present with complex problems
- require more intensive care than normal
- are confused and disoriented
- generally give cause for concern.

Entries should also be made when members of staff provide interventions that affect the degree of:

- risk
- symptomology
- harm
- challenging behaviour
- physical health
- social inclusion.

Courts tend to adopt the attitude that 'if it is not recorded, it has not been done'.

All records can be used as evidence for internal investigations and used in court.

Security, access and confidentiality

An individual's right of access to health records is now governed by the provisions of the Data Protection Act (1998) (DPA) and the Freedom of Information Act (2000). Individuals have the right to access their records in line with local policy and procedure; only information that registered nurses judge could cause serious harm to the physical or mental state of the person, or that would breach the confidentiality of another person can be withheld.

Individuals must be given the opportunity to be involved, as far as is practicable in the circumstances, in planning, developing and reviewing their own treatment and care, to ensure that it is delivered in a way that is appropriate and effective for them.

Individuals have a protected right for their information to be kept in accordance with the DPA and The Caldicott Report (DH, 1997). Information should be kept in confidence – this includes the verbal transmission of information to anybody who is not actively and directly involved in the person's care.

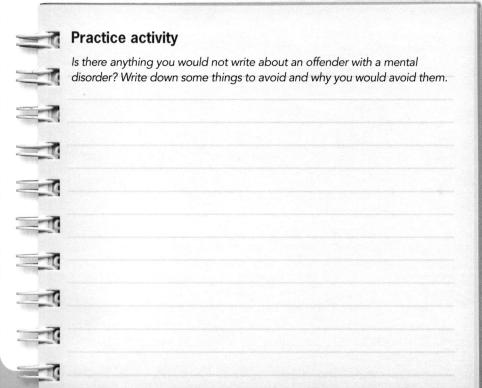

Practice activity

Is there anything you would not write about an offender with a mental disorder? Write down some things to avoid and why you would avoid them.

References

Beck AT, Steer RA & Brown GK (1996) *BDI-II: Beck depression inventory manual*. Boston, MA: Harcourt Brace.

Berne E (1964) *Games People Play*. New York: Grove Press.

Department of Health (1997) *Review on the Review of Patient-identifiable Information (The Caldicott Report)*. London: DH.

Department of Health (2008) *Code of Practice: Mental Health Act 1983*. London: DH.

Department of Health (2010) *Your Guide to Relational Security: See, think, act* [online]. London: Department of Health. Available at: http://www.dh.gov.uk/ prod_consum_dh/groups/dh_digitalassets/documents/digitalasset/dh_113671.pdf (accessed December 2014).

Department of Health (2012) *Winterbourne View Interim Report*. London: DH.

Emerson E (1995) *Challenging Behaviour: Analysis and intervention in people with learning disabilities*. Cambridge: Cambridge University Press.

Mosby's Medical Dictionary (8th edition) (2009) St Louis, MO: Mosby/Elsevier.

Krawiecka M, Goldberg D & Vaughan M (1977) A standardized psychiatric assessment scale for rating chronic psychotic patients. *Acta Psychiatrica Scandinavica* **55** (4) 299–308.

Webster CD, Douglas KS, Eaves D & Hart SD (1997) *HCR-20: Assessing risk for violence* (version 2). Vancouver: Simon Fraser University.

Webster CD, Martin M, Brink J, Nicholls T & Middleton C (2004) *The Short term Assessment of Risk and Treatability (START)*. British Columbia: Forensic Psychiatric Services Commission.

Further reading

Department of Health (2014) *A Positive and Proactive Workforce: A guide to workforce development for commissioners and employers seeking to minimise the use of restrictive practices in social care and health*. London: DH.

Certificate of achievement

This is to certify that:

....

*has achieved xx hours of study and work-based practice on
working in secure forensic mental health settings by covering:*

- *legislation, policies and working with offenders*
- *active support and common mental health problems*
- *assessing risk and recording information.*

Signed: ....

Title: ....

Useful contacts

Care Quality Commission

The CQC checks whether hospitals, care homes, GPs, dentists and services are meeting national standards. It does this by inspecting services and publishing its findings, helping people to make choices about the care they receive.

http://www.cqc.org.uk/

Health Education England

Health Education England (HEE) provides leadership for the new education and training system. It ensures that the workforce has the right skills, behaviours and training, and is available in the right numbers, to support the delivery of excellent healthcare and drive improvements.

http://hee.nhs.uk/

Skills for Care

Skills for Care is the employer-led workforce development body for adult social care in England. It works with employers and other partners to create a fit for purpose qualifications framework and practical resources to develop the skills, knowledge and leadership of the workforce. Its work helps the sector recruit and retain the right people who have the right skills at the right time to deliver high quality services to people who need care and support.

http://www.skillsforcare.org.uk/Home.aspx

Skills for Health

Skills for Health is your sector skills council, for all health employers; NHS, independent and third sector.

http://www.skillsforhealth.org.uk/

Notes